New
Natural Pregnancy

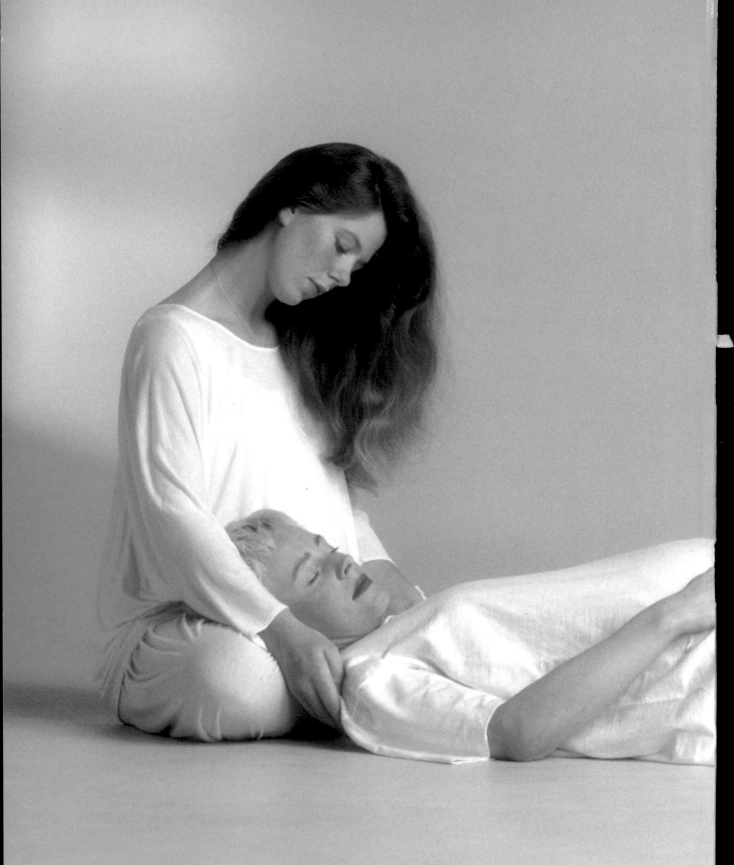

New Natural Pregnancy

Practical wellbeing from conception to birth

Janet Balaskas

Foreword by Yehudi Gordon MD MRCOG FCOGSA

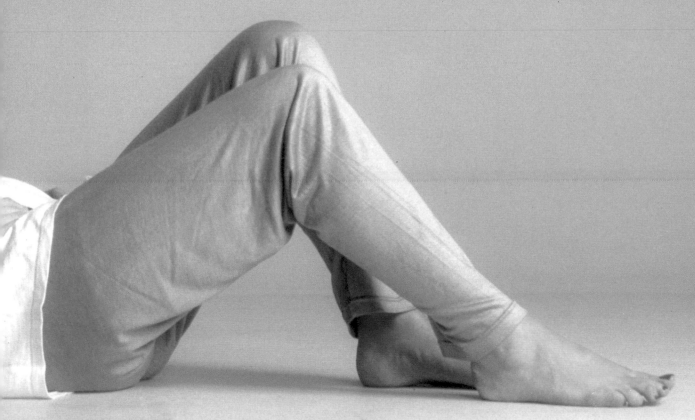

Gaia Books Limited

A GAIA ORIGINAL

Books from Gaia celebrate the vision of Gaia, the self-sustaining living Earth, and seek to help readers live in greater personal and planetary harmony.

Editorial	Helena Petre
Design	Kitty Crossley
Illustration	Lucy Su
Photography	Fausto Dorelli
Additional photography	Steve Teague, Anthea Sieveking, Gus Filgate
Production	Jim Pope
Direction	Patrick Nugent, Jo Godfrey Wood

Published in the United Kingdom by Gaia Books

ISBN 1-85675-219-4
EAN 9781856752190

This is a revised edition of **Natural Pregnancy** (1990)

A catalogue record for this book is available in The British Library

Printed and bound in China

10 9 8 7 6 5 4 3 2 1

Acknowledgements to revised edition
Gaia Books and Janet Balaskas would like to thank the following: Mary Ingoldby for editorial assistance; Anthea Sieveking ; Helen Choules, Penny Robinson, Sarah and Callum Sharp for modelling; Felicity Fine and Juliette Preston for advice on homeopathy and aromatherapy, and Lynn Bresler for proofreading.

Note to the reader
If you are in any doubt about the diagnosis, nature or treatment of a disorder, or if you have had complications during a previous pregnancy, consult your doctor before using the natural therapies in this book.

If X-ray treatment is recommended during the conception period or the early stages of pregnancy, discuss the matter with your doctor.

FOREWORD
TO FIRST EDITION

I am pleased to introduce Janet's book on natural pregnancy. It answers a need for a holistic approach to pregnancy and presents a balanced view of therapies currently available within complementary medicine.

In 1981, Janet coined the term "active birth". She has since become one of the key figures responsible for the new approach to birth philosophy and practice. The Active Birth Movement voices the need felt by parents to be active and take responsibility for their own health and that of their children during pregnancy, at birth, and after birth.

Our health is linked to the health of the planet – worldwide consciousness of the need to protect the environment in which we live is developing rapidly. Governments are under increasing pressure to take stock of our natural resources and to find ways of preserving them for future generations. Every birth, each new baby, has an important role to play. *Natural Pregnancy* is one of many voices currently challenging politicians, doctors, and midwives to respect life's natural flow and to transfer the lessons we are learning from the environment to the needs of individual men, women, and babies as they prepare for birth. Good health, an alert mind, and an open heart clearly help to encourage the natural flow and reduce the need for technological intervention.

The advice on health and gentle healing offered in this book is safe, sensible, and easy to implement. It covers simple holistic techniques and treatments and guides the reader in the search for emotional and spiritual wellbeing, physical fitness, suppleness, and good nutrition. If used under the guidance of a doctor and complementary therapist, *Natural Pregnancy* will help to bridge the gap between conventional and alternative approaches to health.

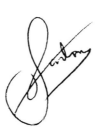

Yehudi Gordon MD MRCOG FCOGSA Consultant Obstetrician

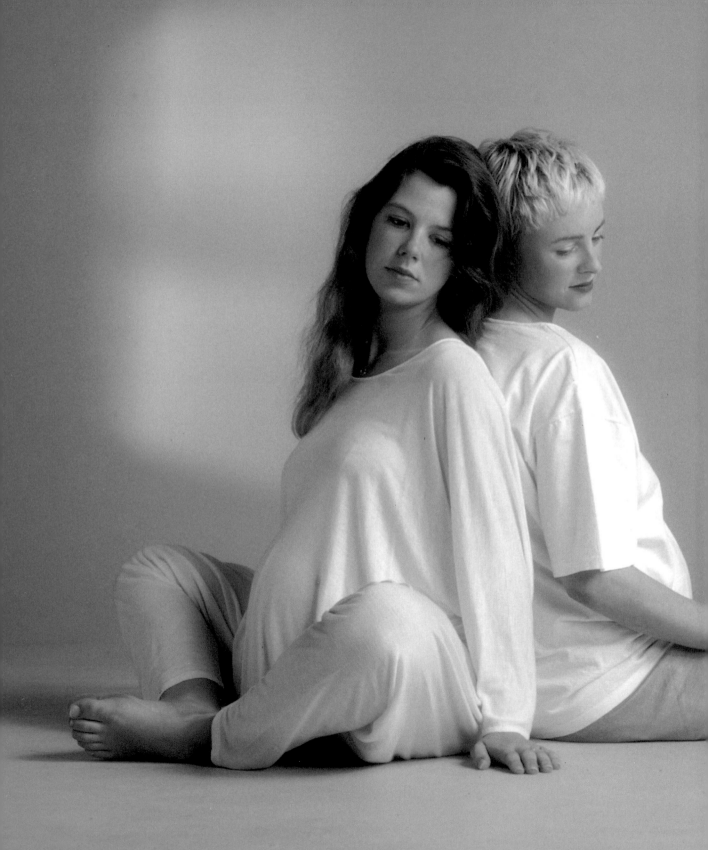

CONTENTS

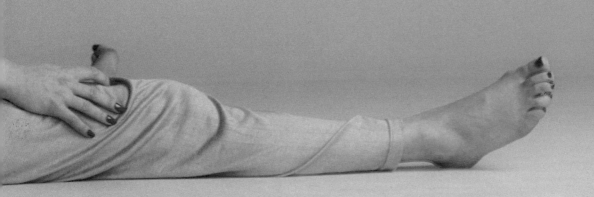

INTRODUCTION

This book is written to help you to take responsibility for your own health and harmony in mind, body, and spirit in the months approaching birth. Its contents will guide and encourage you to discover and develop your inner resources as you prepare for giving birth and being a mother. It is also written to help you to protect and nourish your unborn child and to make the most of your potential for influencing his or her development positively before the birth.

Following the invention of forceps in the 17th century, birth in the West increasingly came under the control of doctors. Women gradually lost contact with their own power and potential for giving birth as first the passive reclining position and then the use of anaesthesia became widespread. As a logical sequence, the art of breastfeeding declined and bottle-feeding of babies became the norm. During this time pregnancy itself was regarded as a semi-invalid state. Pregnant women were surrounded by taboos and old wives' tales, and birth became primarily a medical event.

Thankfully, there has been a rebellion against this sort of attitude. Today, pregnancy is seen as a normal, healthy event and there is a growing trend all over the world toward natural, active childbirth and breastfeeding. However, prenatal care is still "patient" orientated and primarily concerned with medical checking and screening for possible problems. There is rarely any time given to taking an interest in your emotional life, let alone to helping you maximize your health and wellbeing. No-one will deny that modern obstetrics is invaluable when difficulties or problems do arise, but many women are questioning the routine use of intervention or medication and are looking for other more natural ways to promote a trouble-free pregnancy and birth. In the years to come, women can expect to have a much greater freedom to choose from a range of alternatives within the maternity services. Appropriate care in pregnancy, while using the benefits of science (when necessary) will also place greater emphasis on complementary therapies, good nutrition, and exercise. As the importance of the relationship between the pregnant mother and her midwife is more widely recognised, the ancient healing arts traditionally associated with midwifery will be brought to life.

New Natural Pregnancy offers a holistic approach to pregnancy that aims to help you increase your self-reliance and confidence by encouraging you to prepare physically, emotionally, and spiritually during the nine months before you give birth. The first chapter contains advice on how to cope with the emotional challenges of pregnancy and how to calm and centre yourself through deep breathing and meditation. Subsequent chapters give clear, practical guidelines on achieving health during pregnancy. They cover the fundamentals of a wholesome, nutritious diet and give step-by-step instructions for practising basic yoga and massage sequences, which will deepen your physical awareness and help you to trust in the miraculous processes of birth and breastfeeding. This body-orientated way of preparing for birth has evolved over the years I have spent working with pregnant women who come to the Active Birth Centre in London. It is also based on my experiences during my own pregnancies and the births of my four children. Theo, the youngest, was born at home a few months before I began to write this book. He weighed in at 5kg (11lb) and, despite the fact that I am now over 40, was born like his brother and two sisters without complications, thanks to a natural pregnancy.

Regular practice of meditation, yoga, and massage is the best way to prepare yourself for birth and motherhood. It will bring your mind and body into a healthy union, and is far more empowering and effective in helping you to achieve a natural, active birth than acquiring a lot of theoretical information or learning complicated breathing methods.

The two final chapters describe natural, or alternative, therapies and how they can be used safely and effectively to maintain and restore health during pregnancy. Many of the common ailments that may occur in pregnancy are covered, together with reliable guidelines for prevention, self-help, and professional treatment using natural therapies.

At the Active Birth Centre I work in association with a number of alternative practitioners who use natural therapies to treat emotional problems and physical discomforts experienced by pregnant women. I have seen the powerful healing effects that these therapies can have without endangering mother or baby in any way. They can very often bring relief to specific problems for which orthodox medicine has little to offer.

I hope that this book will help you to enjoy and make the most of your pregnancy. Knowing how best to maintain your own health through exercise and massage can make a tremendous difference to the way you feel.

When appropriately used, natural therapies will help you to maximize your inner potential for health. They will also increase your sense of power and responsibility and awaken your motherly instinct for healing your baby naturally after the birth. I hope that you will be encouraged to take advantage of the great benefits that natural therapies have to offer you at this time, and that this book will help to stimulate a change to a more holistic approach to prenatal care.

CHAPTER 1

EMOTIONS

During pregnancy you will be preparing both emotionally and physically to meet the challenges of birth and motherhood. From an early stage you will probably find that your feelings tend to surface more easily. You may experience rapid changes of mood, laugh and cry more than usual, become angry more directly and audibly, and be generally less in control of your emotions than you were. Having your feelings so close to the surface can be frightening but it also means that they are more accessible, and that you have the opportunity for change and transformation if you are willing to feel and express them.

Your reaction to confirmation of the pregnancy will depend on your circumstances. If the pregnancy was intentional, you may be radiant with happiness, excitement, and joy. If, on the other hand, conception was accidental, the news may come as a surprise, or even a shock, and may involve considerable adjustment.

No matter what your circumstances, coming to terms with pregnancy may take time and the early months are usually accompanied by a wide range of feelings. Some women also experience tiredness and nausea, while others feel well and energetic. By the end of the third month, however, things generally settle down. Feelings of apprehension may still occur from time to time but these should soon subside, leaving you feeling more relaxed and confident, and able to look forward to the time ahead. At around 18 weeks, your belly will begin to show and sometime in the following two weeks you should experience the first flutterings of sensation as your baby starts to move. This is the time to celebrate and enjoy the rounded sensuality of your body — to do yoga, to swim, to be massaged, and to relax out of doors in natural surroundings. Caring for yourself, and spending time on activities that enhance your peace of mind, self-confidence, and health will all help to nourish your baby.

Throughout your pregnancy powerful protective feelings for your child will be developing. And as you approach birth, your nesting instinct will arise most strongly. Physically, you may feel bursts of energy accompanied by a need to slow down and rest. It is natural for the more mental faculties such as intellect and memory to quiet down temporarily during pregnancy while your instincts and intuition become stronger. This is even more true toward the end as you await the day that labour starts and look forward to the excitement and joy of welcoming your new baby.

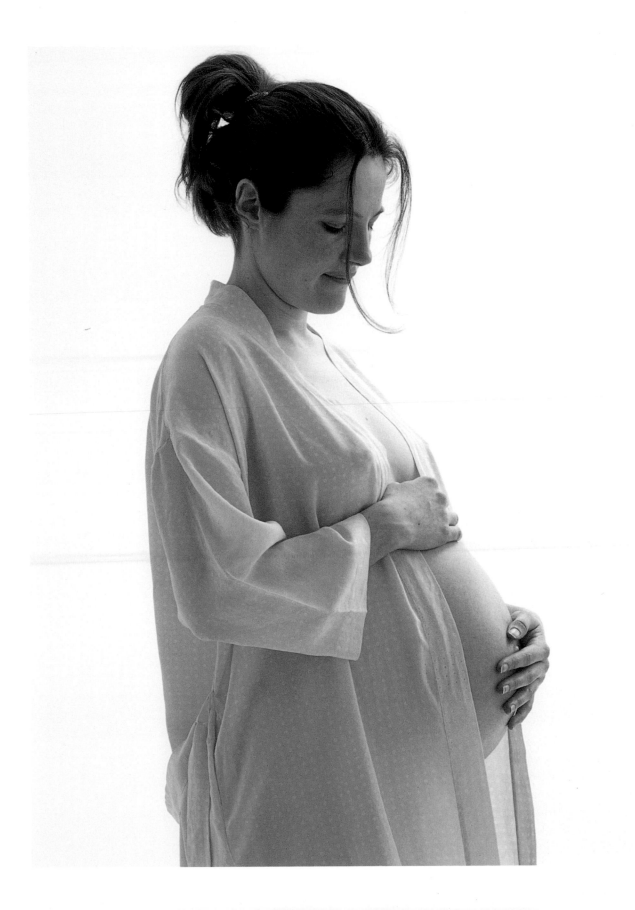

Clearing the past

While not everyone needs to do so, pregnancy can be a good time to clear up any unresolved emotional issues from your past. You can begin by taking a look at your early life, and at what was happening around the time of your own conception, gestation period, and birth, as well as recalling the formative years of your infancy and childhood.

Your relationship with your parents, especially your mother, take on a new relevance as you approach parenthood yourself. While some people are fortunate enough to have had a happy childhood and a satisfactory relationship with their parents, for others the opposite may be true or there may have been some tragedy in their lives, the loss of someone close to them, or some other traumatic experience. Many people have an unconscious tendency to repeat patterns from the past in present relationships. Part of the process of maturing is to become conscious of these patterns through placing your own childhood and parenting in perspective, and thus to have the freedom and self-awareness to change them if you choose to. It will help to look at family attitudes and beliefs about sex, pregnancy, and birth, and to explore any issues about which you are unhappy or fearful. This can be done by verbal sharing with a partner, friend or therapist, or on your own, by writing your feelings down, meditating, or in any other way that works for you. Try to release your emotions fully – to cry away grief, and to feel and express any anger, fear, disgust, or jealousy, particularly if it has been held down in the past. If you have had a miscarriage or termination/abortion, are troubled by memories of a previous birth, or have suffered sexual abuse, it is important to acknowledge any buried or painful feelings relating to this experience.

Dreams tend to be more vivid in pregnancy and provide a medium through which your unconscious desires and anxieties can surface. Writing your dreams down as soon as you wake up can be a further aid to exploring your inner world.

If you have many painful feelings to work through, you may fear that doing so in pregnancy will harm your baby. Since these feelings exist inside you anyway, it will be an advantage to you both to release them and to clear the way to enjoyable motherhood. If, however, you find it difficult to get in touch or cope with your emotions, or feel depressed or frequently anxious, it is important to seek help, consulting a therapist if necessary (see p. 67). When you give birth you will find it easier to let go if you are not attempting to control or suppress your feelings. Postnatal/postpartum depression is also less likely to occur if you have been able to release any deeply buried feelings during pregnancy.

When exploring your past, it is important also to acknowledge the good things, and to feel confident that all the love and nourishment you received as a child, as well as the difficult and painful times, have prepared you well for the challenges of motherhood. Whatever your circumstances, coming to terms with the truth is an opportunity for self-discovery and personal development. It will free you to enjoy the bliss and euphoria that are part of having a baby, and to find your way as a parent.

Anticipating the birth

Toward the end of pregnancy, life may become more emotionally demanding. Faced with the realities of the approaching birth and motherhood, you may at times experience anxiety, fear, or even occasional panic. Physically, you may feel less comfortable and find it difficult to sleep sometimes. It is quite natural at this stage to have doubts about your ability to cope with pain in labour or whether you can manage to give birth or produce a perfect baby.

Acknowledging and expressing these fears is one way to overcome them. It is also important to gain an understanding of the physiological processes of birth (see *Further Reading,* p. 93) and to familiarize yourself with obstetric back-up procedures, so that you are aware of what can be done if difficulties do arise. Attending prenatal yoga classes will help you to develop confidence and trust in your body and your natural ability to give birth.

Becoming a mother

Like anything truly worthwhile, becoming a mother is a profoundly challenging experience. During the first few years your baby will be totally dependent on you and you will need to come to terms with the responsibility that parenting entails. Since the way that you respond to your baby is vital to his or her happiness and health, it may be reassuring to know that most of us, given realistic expectations, learn to be good enough mothers.

Many women, however, underestimate the sheer hard work, dedication, and patience involved in caring for a baby. Spending time with other mothers and their babies while you are pregnant will help to prepare you. It is also a good idea to give some preliminary thought to feeding and caring for your baby after the birth.

In many ways, however, nothing can prepare you in advance for motherhood. You may, for example, be surprised by the intensity of the love you feel for your baby, while at other times feelings of anger and despair may be uppermost. Fulfilling your baby's needs will have to be your priority for some time after the birth, but there will be unique and wonderful moments when your love is spontaneously returned. It is at these times that you will experience the elation and sense of fulfilment that make all the work involved in mothering worthwhile.

If through circumstances or choice you are facing the transition to motherhood on your own, it is important to find someone in whom you can confide, and to plan your life so that you have as much support, friendship, and nurturing as possible. Seek out the company of other pregnant women and make the effort to attend yoga or birth-preparation classes. You can invite a friend or relative to accompany you, and also perhaps arrange for someone to be with you at the birth. Plan well for the postnatal period, finding out ahead of time whether or not you are entitled to financial help after the birth. You can also try contacting a single parent association (see *Useful Addresses,* p. 93).

Family relationships

Before you begin the shared adventure of parenthood, it is important to consolidate and strengthen your relationship with your partner. The nine months ahead will give you the opportunity to sort out any unresolved conflicts and to agree on your long-term goals in having a child as well as the way in which you intend to care for your baby. Make the most of this time to work on your communication, so that you learn how to share your feelings and to listen to each other.

While you may become increasingly conscious of the child that you are carrying inside you, your partner may not have the same awareness, and may need to be encouraged to focus on the pregnancy and to participate in pre-natal care, massage, and birth-preparation classes. He can offer you great reassurance and emotional support if he is ready to be actively involved, and this can extend into sharing the birth experience and parenthood. After the birth, much of your time will be taken up with the baby and your partner will need both to adapt to the inevitable temporary neglect that is the new father's lot, and to nurture you both for a while in a way that he may not be used to. In addition, he may have new challenges at work or additional financial responsibilities. The strains and stress that fathers experience are not usually socially recognized, and it will help if you can try to be aware of what your partner is going through, and make an effort to spend a quiet period together from time to time. A useful exercise is to sit down facing each other when you have a quiet moment. Start by breathing deeply and simply looking into each other's eyes for a few minutes in silence. Then take turns to tell each other how you are feeling. Allow your partner to speak while you listen without comment, and then exchange roles. If you feel uncomfortable doing this exercise, then try to set aside time to talk. Being a good listener and sensitive to your partner's needs is the way to enjoy parenting as a team and to meet its challenges from a calm, united centre.

If this is a second or subsequent pregnancy, you will have the additional challenge of integrating the new baby into your present family. Other children, especially younger ones, are bound to feel some pain as the new baby becomes the focus for your attention, taking up most of your time and energy at first. They will need careful and sensitive preparation if they are to come to terms with and accept the new arrival. You can help by reassuring the older child that he or she is loved and by planning to be together as much as possible in the first few days after the birth.

Make time to introduce your unborn child gradually to other members of the family. Encourage your older child to become familiar with the unborn baby through massage, watching his or her movements, guessing where the head, arms, and legs are, or listening to the heartbeat during a check-up. At the same time, try to expand the older child's horizons and encourage close relationships with your partner, or with another relative or helper. Above all, try to be understanding when he or she is releasing feelings or being rather difficult or babyish – this type of reaction is to be expected alongside the enthusiasm and love that he or she is bound to feel for the new baby.

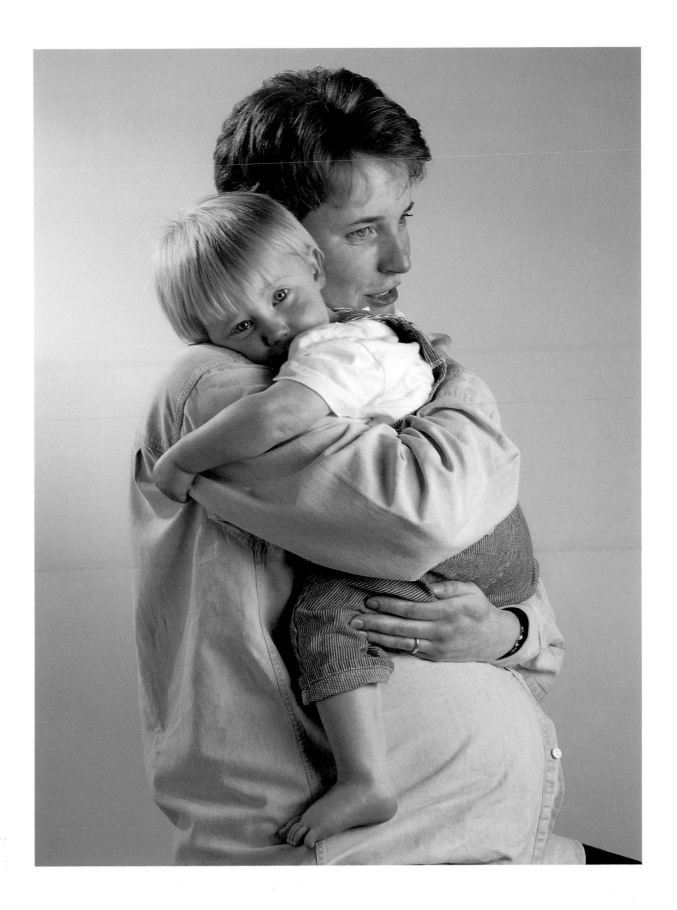

Lovemaking

Making love is the instinctive expression of affection that brings our bodies into contact and our souls into harmony. It is also an act of creation in which a new life may be formed.

Some couples are conscious of their desire to have a child and the intention to start a pregnancy can heighten lovemaking in a very special way. Often, however, conception is unplanned but can be celebrated by sexuality during pregnancy. This is a time when you and your partner will be consolidating your relationship and will need both to give and receive more love and affection, and to be held, caressed, and reassured. Now, even more than at other times, intimacy, mutual tenderness, respect, and consideration for each other's needs are important.

As a starting point, it is good to know that it's perfectly safe to make love during pregnancy. The developing foetus is well protected by the amniotic fluid and the membranes, and deep penetration, if your partner is gentle, will not harm the baby since your uterus is situated well above the vagina. Occasionally making love can cause spotting because the blood vessels around the cervix are more plentiful during pregnancy and some of them may rupture. This is not usually a cause for concern, but it is wise, nevertheless, to inform your doctor, who may recommend that you avoid deep penetration for a short period. It is unlikely that making love could cause a miscarriage, but women with a tendency to miscarry are often advised to avoid full sexual contact for the first 12 weeks until pregnancy is well established.

Sexuality during pregnancy

Many women find pregnancy a sexual and erotic time and may even experience full orgasm for the first time. Ironically, it is the one time when you can make love with abandon and without any need for contraception.

Experiencing orgasm is perfectly safe, and probably beneficial in tonifying the uterus and preparing your body for birth, which is in itself an orgasmic release. The period of blissful relaxation that may follow orgasm is calming and energizing and will produce a glowing love-energy for your baby. You may find that your uterus remains hard and firm for some minutes afterward. This is quite normal and similar in effect to the practice, or Braxton Hicks, contractions that you experience toward the end of your pregnancy as your uterus prepares for birth.

Some women experience a lessening of desire for intercourse in pregnancy, especially in the early months when they may feel vulnerable or be suffering from tiredness or nausea. These feelings often pass by mid term but may recur in the final weeks approaching birth when the weight of the heavy uterus can cause some discomfort. A complete loss of desire for sex during pregnancy is also not uncommon and is quite normal. If, however, you feel you have a deeper inhibition, a history of frigidity, or difficulty achieving orgasm, then it may be advisable to consult a psychotherapist or a sex-therapist. The source of the problem may lie in your relationship with your partner, in which case it is vital to try and sort it out to prevent unnecessary stress both prior to, during, and after the birth. One or both of you may have unwarranted fears that love-making will injure, harm, or disturb the baby, and you may both find it helpful to discuss the subject. You may, for example, feel concerned that your baby could be emotionally upset by lovemaking. Provided both partners are enjoying the experience and movements are gentle, this is unlikely. It may even be positively beneficial for your baby to be surrounded by the warmth, affection, and bliss that are all part of making love. Alternatively, you may be worried that intercourse will start premature labour, but this will not occur unless you are on the brink of giving birth anyway, in which case lovemaking may help to bring labour on. If you are overdue, you may find that intercourse will stimulate the start of labour since a hormone in semen called prostaglandin helps to soften the cervix – a natural preparation for birth!

Comfortable positions

Pregnancy is the perfect time to explore different positions for making love. Indeed, from mid pregnancy onwards as your belly expands, you will need to take care to avoid resting your weight on your baby. Make sure you have plenty of soft pillows around to make yourself comfortable. You can try lying on your side with your partner behind you, or adopt a kneeling position like the one used in the pelvic release exercise on page 38, position c, with your partner lying on his back underneath you. This latter position will allow you to control the depth of penetration. Another possibility is for you to kneel comfortably on all fours over a pile of cushions and for your partner to enter from behind. Allow yourself to be inventive and communicate openly with your partner so that you both feel able to give the honest feedback necessary in satisfying lovemaking.

There are no rules in making love and during pregnancy there may be times when full intercourse is not appropriate. Oral sex is often enjoyed during this period and it is useful to know that the tissues of the vagina may become fuller in pregnancy, and that secretions increase so the normal taste and feel of your genital area may be different. Massaging each other with an aromatic oil is a way of making love with your hands. Nipple massage and stimulation is, in fact, the best possible way to prepare your breasts for breast-feeding. It is also perfectly safe and normal to masturbate, especially if you are alone or if your partner does not feel like full intercourse. It is in any case helpful to feel comfortable and familiar with your own genital area before giving birth.

Making love is a close and intimate communication and your inner harmony depends on your feeling at ease with your physical self and uninhibited about your natural urges. Pregnancy is the perfect time to enjoy the sensuality of your body without guilt and to make the most of the potential for deepening your relationship with your partner, in readiness to include your child in the love you share. The feeling of oneness experienced during and after lovemaking helps to nourish body and soul and is a natural expression of the love that forms the basis of family life.

Breathing

Breathing is essential to life and is the key to health, harmony, and peace of mind. While you are pregnant and during labour, you are breathing for yourself and also for your baby, so it is important to ensure that you are breathing well. Spending a little time each day practising deep breathing and focusing your awareness on your breath will help you to find your inner centre and to calm yourself to make the most of the good times, and to use your resources to cope with any difficulties that may arise. Deep breathing also brings your body into harmony with gravity, making you feel grounded (see p. 32) and enabling you to release tension. This is important when practising yoga (see pp. 30-43) and during strong contractions in labour. You do not need to learn any special breathing techniques for the birth. Simply cultivate the habit of breathing deeply when you meditate, practise your yoga, or give or receive a massage, and you will learn to do so spontaneously in labour, in harmony with the natural movements of your body.

Practise the exercise described daily if you can in a well-ventilated room or outside. Sit comfortably on the floor, supporting your lower back against a wall if necessary. Fold your legs (see opposite), cross them, or sit with them comfortably stretched out in front of you.

Deep breathing exercise

Close your eyes and concentrate on your breathing. As you exhale, relax your whole body. Let your pelvis settle securely on the ground by releasing your lower back toward the floor. Lengthen the back of your neck by letting your chin drop slightly toward your chest. Release your shoulders downward and relax your abdomen and pelvic floor. Place your palms on your lower belly and observe the rhythm of your breathing. When you are ready, begin to focus on the exhalations, breathing out slowly through your mouth, and in gently through your nose.

Sense the exhalation as if it were starting at the top of your spine and moving down the column of vertebrae to your tailbone. From there, feel the outward breath continuing downward as if it were sending roots deep into the earth below your sitting bones. At the same time, feel how your belly empties away from your hands as the pressure in your abdomen decreases. Pause for a second. Now inhale slowly, still aware of the grounded feeling in your pelvis. Allow the breath to come in lightly and effortlessly of its own accord. Sense the inhalation rising from the deep roots and travelling all the way up your spine to the base of the skull, creating space and lightness. At the same time, feel how your belly expands toward your hands as pressure in the abdomen increases. Continue breathing in this way, feeling the waves of inward and outward breath caress the spine with a smooth and natural rhythm. You should be able to feel the fluctuating movement of the breath in the abdomen with your hands, while your chest remains calm and still. After 5 to 10 minutes, place your hands palms up on your knees. Focus on the wave of your breathing and sit in silence for a while.

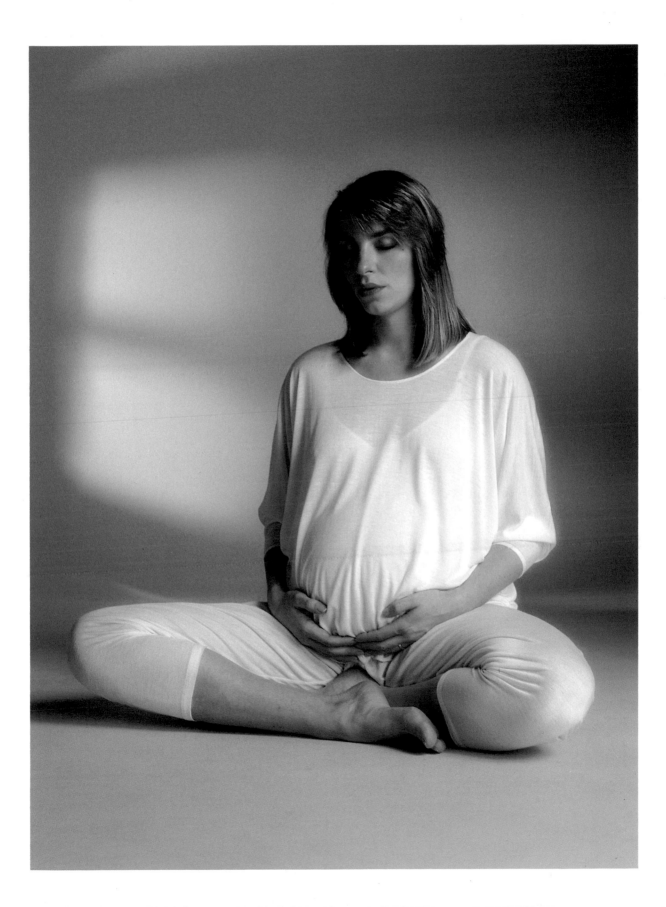

Chakra meditation

In the yogic tradition, our sexual energy, known as *kundalini-shakti*, is seen as a coiled serpent that lies at the base of the spine and rises up through the body toward the head. As it rises, it passes through the subtle energy centres, or *chakras*, each of which is associated with a sound and a colour. Meditation on the chakras arouses the kundalini energy and cleanses and clears the subtle energy centres. It is both energizing and relaxing, and a powerful and agreeable way to release tension during pregnancy. It also prepares you to release sound spontaneously and without inhibition when giving birth.

To prepare yourself for meditation, follow the instructions given on page 18 for deep breathing. Once you are comfortably relaxed, start with the base chakra in the pelvis (see below), releasing the sound *OOO* (as in you) along with the exhalation. Feel the sound coming from deep down in your pelvis and take it to the very end of the breath; then pause and let the inhalation come in freely. Repeat this a few more times, and as you release the sound, visualize red light emanating from the centre of your pelvic area and radiating outward. Following the diagram, work your way up through the different energy centres, using the appropriate sounds and colours, until you reach the crown chakra. This is described as a thousand-petalled lotus that opens toward the divine energy of the universe, uplifting the spirit toward ecstasy and bliss. End the meditation by chanting the sound *OM* three times and sitting in silence.

During pregnancy work with the six chakras illustrated to harmonize your whole being. Breathing deeply, chant the sound of the chakra when you exhale, taking the sound to the end of the breath, then inhale slowly and repeat several times. Visualize the chakra as a spinning sphere with coloured light radiating out from the centre together with the sound vibration. For inspiration, use crayons to colour in the illustrated chakras.

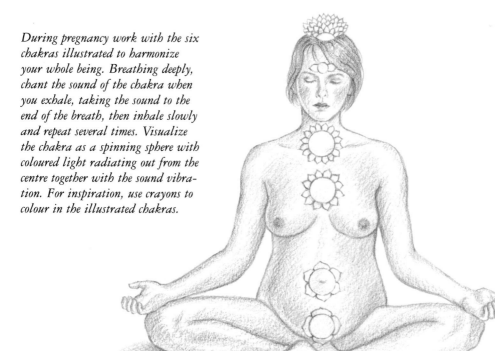

Crown
Thousand-petalled Lotus
Sound: OM
Colour: Pure white light

Third eye
Sound: EEE (as in bee)
Colour: Violet

Throat
Sound: EH (as in egg)
Colour: Indigo blue

Heart
Sound: AAH (as in far)
Colour: Brilliant green

Navel
Sound: AW (as in saw)
Colour: Yellow

Base
Sexual Energy
Sound OOO (as in you)
Colour: Red

Baby meditation

In ancient China and Japan, pregnant women were encouraged to practise meditation daily and to communicate with their babies during pregnancy in the following way. Sit comfortably with your eyes closed. Breathe deeply and relax, allowing yourself to become quiet, calm and centred (see p. 18), and to focus inwardly on the presence of your baby. Taking your time, visualize your baby's tiny body – the head, arms, legs, and even the fingers and toes – perfectly formed inside your womb. See if you can tune in to the consciousness of your unborn child and imagine what he or she is experiencing. Imagine how the warm amniotic fluid must feel on the sensitive surface of your baby's skin and what it must be like to move and somersault free from the effects of gravity. Imagine the sounds that your baby hears – your voice, the reassuring regularity of your heartbeat, and the gentle rumblings of your digestive system. Your baby may also be able to hear music, voices, and other sounds from outside the womb.

The psychic and emotional connection between you is established long before birth so that your moods, feelings, and even dreams may enter the consciousness of your unborn child. This is not to say that negative feelings may be harmful, but only that while meditating you can consciously communicate with and send loving messages to your baby. Spend some time just being with your baby and then open your eyes, retaining an inner awareness of your child's presence as you return to your daily activities. Meditate in this way for a few minutes every day, if you can.

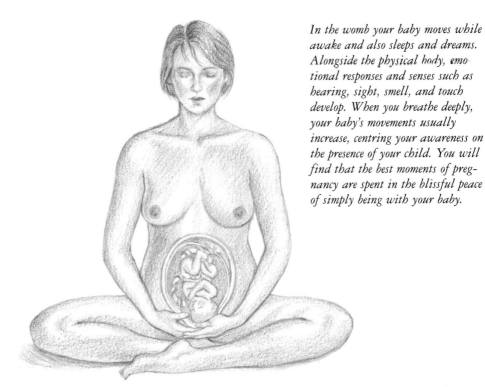

In the womb your baby moves while awake and also sleeps and dreams. Alongside the physical body, emotional responses and senses such as hearing, sight, smell, and touch develop. When you breathe deeply, your baby's movements usually increase, centring your awareness on the presence of your child. You will find that the best moments of pregnancy are spent in the blissful peace of simply being with your baby.

CHAPTER 2

NUTRITION

During pregnancy all the essential nutrients your baby needs pass through the placenta from your bloodstream. While your own circulation and that of the developing baby remain quite separate, you continue to breathe, eat, and excrete for your baby throughout pregnancy and labour until the placenta is delivered after the birth. A nutritious, balanced diet is thus vitally important during this period, both for your own health and for that of your growing baby. Eating the right foods will give your baby a good start in life, as well as enabling you to maintain good energy throughout pregnancy, birth, and during the postnatal period.

Whether you eat animal foods or are vegetarian or vegan, you will be able to use the information on the following pages to achieve a healthy diet. Concentrate on improving the quality and variety of your diet to ensure that you have all the raw materials that you need.

If you ate well before becoming pregnant, you should have sufficient reserves to cope with any periods of deficiency that may occur if, for example, nausea makes it difficult to eat properly for a while. An inadequate diet, however, can leave your reserves depleted and, while your baby may be able to obtain all the nutrients that he or she requires, you may be left with an insufficient supply for your own needs.

For this reason, it is essential that your daily intake of proteins, fats, carbohydrates, vitamins, and minerals is correctly balanced, and made up of fresh wholesome foods. Eating well will also reduce the likelihood of complications arising during pregnancy and birth.

To help develop healthy nutritional habits, bear in mind these simple points: always keep your kitchen clean and dry, and wash your hands before preparing food. Defrost frozen food thoroughly, and never exceed the "use by" date on food, even if it looks perfectly edible. Cook red meat, chicken, fish, and eggs thoroughly. Keep the fridge temperature below 5 degrees C and the freezer below -18 degrees C. Where possible, eat organic produce.

Combining good nutrition with regular exercise (see pp. 30-43) will give you added strength and energy as well as helping to ensure your rapid recovery during the postnatal period.

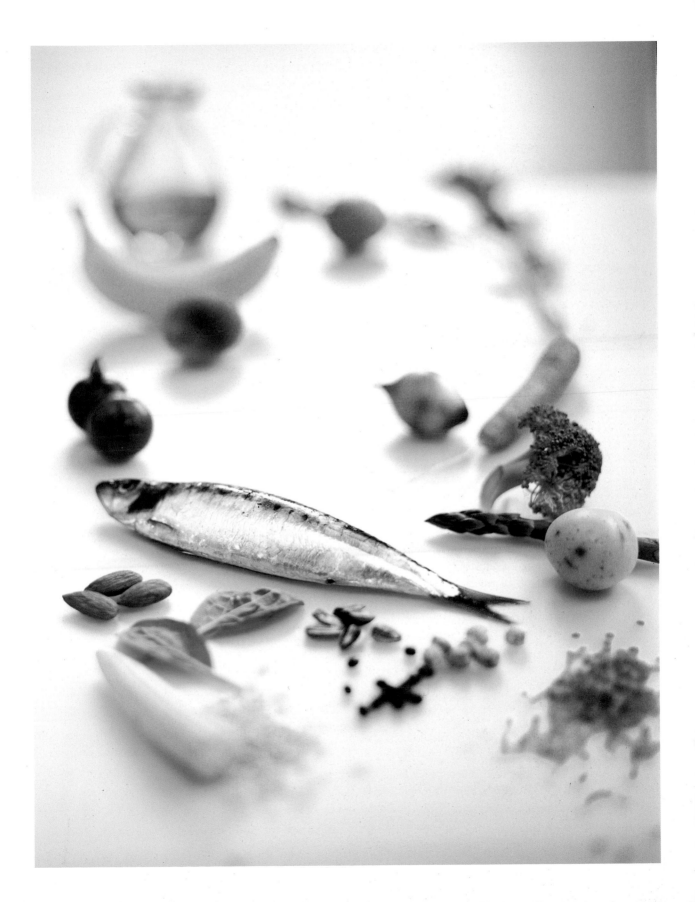

Selecting fresh, wholesome foods

Eating well enough to maintain your health and nourish your baby should not be difficult, provided you choose a suitably varied selection of foods and eat unrefined, fresh produce whenever possible.

Include fresh fruit, vegetables, and salads in your daily diet and buy fresh meat or fish in preference to using packaged or frozen varieties. It is best to buy mainly fresh produce because many of the processes used to preserve foods, such as freezing and canning, result in a loss of nutrients. Try to choose local, freshly picked fruit and vegetables since nutrients may be lost during lengthy storage. It is also important to read labels carefully and avoid products that contain flavouring, colourings, and preservatives, since these can be harmful to both your own and your baby's health. Some processed wholefood products, however, are highly nutritious and contain no chemicals. Preserved organic soya bean products, such as tofu, tempeh, miso and tamari, for example, are high in protein, iron, calcium, and B vitamins and are a good substitute for meat. Yeast extract, cold pressed oils, honey, and farmhouse cheeses are other examples of nutritious processed foods.

Try whenever possible to eat whole rather than refined foods. Parts of the food are removed during the refining process and vital nutrients and natural fibre are lost. The result is a product with a reduced nutritional value and one that is less easily digested since natural fibre aids the processes of digestion and elimination. To increase the wholefood content of your diet, buy wholegrain bread and brown rather than white rice, since the former retains its outer husks. You can eat organically grown fruit and vegetables unpeeeled but, where pesticides have been used, either remove the skin or scrub the surface area thoroughly.

Many wholefood beans and grains are wonderfully nutritious when sprouted, containing proteins, fats, carbohydrates, fibre, vitamins, minerals, and trace elements. If you sprout the seeds yourself and eat them in salads and sandwiches or stir-fries soon after they germinate, the "live" nutrients they contain are particularly easy to assimilate. Experiment with mung beans, soya beans, aduki beans, lentils, wholewheat grains, chick peas, or alfalfa seeds, using a sprouter available from a health-food store.

In recent years many doubts have been raised about intensive farming methods and the use of antibiotics in animal farming. While meat is highly nutritious, only organically reared beef, lamb, and chicken from a reputable source can be regarded as free of harmful additives. Liver is best avoided, since it is high in vitamin A. Fish can be eaten regularly, though high sea fish (see *B complex vitamins*, p. 25) are considered less polluted than freshwater fish.

Organic vegetables, fruit, and grains, produced without the use of chemical fertilizers and pesticides, are now more widely available and it is certainly worth trying to find a supplier in your area. Likewise, try to find a local source of organic eggs, poultry, and meat that have not been subjected to growth hormones or antibiotics. You can balance the extra expense by eating meat less frequently; beans or grains make a nutritious substitute and can be bought cheaply in bulk.

Essential nutrients

Proteins, fats, carbohydrates, vitamins, and minerals are the basic ingredients of a healthy diet. Any one food may contain several of these essential nutrients, together with the substances needed to assist their absorption.

Proteins provide essential amino acids for building new tissues as well as ensuring that enzymes, hormones, and antibodies are able to function effectively. During pregnancy you need more protein foods than usual so it is important to be aware of your daily intake. Meat, fish, poultry, dairy products, and eggs provide complete, or first-class, proteins that are easily assimilated, whereas beans and nuts contain "limiting amino acids" which need to be eaten with grains in order for the body to obtain enough protein. Organic soya beans provide the most complete source of vegetable protein.

Fats are a prime source of energy and ensure the smooth functioning of the body, in particular the nervous system. They contain the vitamins A and D, and are found in meat, fish, dairy products, and vegetable oils.

Carbohydrates are made up of sugars, starch, and fibre, and are a major source of energy. They are found in potatoes, grains, and beans.

Vitamins and minerals are essential for healthy growth and development. Eating a wide variety of fresh, whole produce will provide you with the best supply of these vital nutrients since certain vitamins are found in highest concentration beneath the skins of fruit and vegetables; others, especially vitamin C, are easily destroyed by cooking or processing.

Important vitamins and minerals in pregnancy

Iron Iron is an essential ingredient of haemoglobin, the substance in your blood that carries oxygen to your baby. As much as one third of your iron intake is used by your baby to make blood and build up stores for after the birth. *Sources* beef, sardines, eggs, dried fruit (especially figs, prunes, raisins, and apricots), almonds, black strap molasses, brewer's yeast, cocoa, wholegrain bread, sprouted seeds and grains, beetroot/beets, broccoli, green leafy vegetables, seaweeds.

Combine iron-rich foods with vitamin C to aid iron absorption. Avoid drinking tea or coffee with or immediately after meals since these stimulants inhibit iron absorption.

Folic acid During pregnancy you need twice as much folic acid as usual to assist the use of iron, to help build red blood cells, and to develop your baby's nervous system. *Sources* Dark leafy greens, broccoli, spinach, brewer's yeast, root vegetables, whole and sprouted grains, oysters, salmon, whole milk, dates, and mushrooms.

Vitamin C A natural antibiotic, vitamin C helps to fight and prevent infection as well as assisting absorption of iron. *Sources* Citrus fruits, strawberries, blackcurrants, raspberries, watermelon, kiwi fruits, broccoli, Brussels sprouts, potatoes, and cabbage.

Zinc This mineral promotes growth and healing and may help prevent nausea. *Sources* oysters, seafood, nuts, carrots, sweetcorn, tomatoes, bananas, brewer's yeast, wholegrain, and sprouted seeds, grains, and meat.

Calcium A natural tranquillizer, calcium ensures the normal functioning of nerves and muscles and is also essential for strong bones and teeth. *Sources* Dairy products, salmon, sardines, organic soya beans, brewer's yeast, sesame seeds, almonds, sprouted seeds and grains, seaweed, collard greens, and kale.

B complex vitamins These vitamins perform essential functions in the body. *Sources* Yeast, eggs, organic soya beans, high sea fish such as mackerel and sardines, wheatgerm, avocados, nuts, and sunflower seeds.

Combining and balancing foods

In pregnancy your daily diet should contain approximately 40 per cent cereal foods, 25 per cent vegetables, 30 per cent proteins, and 5 per cent fresh and dried fruit. To ensure a good balance, combine foods that you like from the four basic groups illustrated below when making up your daily menus. Use the recommended number of portions as a guide. Individual portions should weigh between 85 and 170g (3-6oz).

Protein foods

Proteins are found in meat, fish, poultry, eggs, beans, peas, lentils, nuts, and seeds. All types of meat are rich in protein, particularly organ meats, which also have a high concentration of vitamins and minerals, while eggs are a well-balanced source of protein. Fish contains both proteins and unsaturated fats, so make good use of the wide range available, including both white and oily brown types. You will find non-animal protein in lentils, black-eyed beans, chick peas, soya beans, haricot beans, lima beans, and mung beans. Organic soya beans are an excellent source of complete vegetable protein, but other beans need to be eaten with grains (see p. 25). Include almonds, brazil nuts, hazelnuts, walnuts, cashews, and lightly roasted sunflower, sesame, or pumpkin seeds. Aim to eat 2-3 portions per day of protein foods.

Cereal foods

Cereals are full of the carbohydrates our bodies need for energy and they are also a rich source of protein, fibre, and essential minerals and vitamins. You can include cereals in your diet by eating porridge, muesli, wholegrain cereals or bread, and wholewheat couscous or pasta. You should eat 4-6 servings of a cereal food per day.

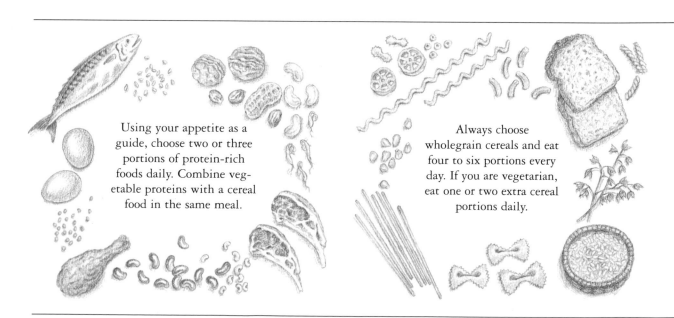

Using your appetite as a guide, choose two or three portions of protein-rich foods daily. Combine vegetable proteins with a cereal food in the same meal.

Always choose wholegrain cereals and eat four to six portions every day. If you are vegetarian, eat one or two extra cereal portions daily.

Vegetables and fruit

Vegetables and fruit play important roles in a wholefood diet and you should try to eat a varied selection each week in order to be sure of getting enough of the different minerals, vitamins, oils, and fibres that they contain. Use unpeeled organic vegetables whenever possible, scrubbing the skins clean with a brush. To retain their nutritional value, lightly steam, stir fry, or bake them, so that they remain slightly crunchy. Always peel vegetables that are not organic. Leafy green vegetables are particularly beneficial in pregnancy since they contain both iron and folic acid (see p. 25). Include nutrient-rich seaweeds (see p. 28), and try to eat a raw, fresh salad daily.

Fruits contain many vitamins and minerals, notably vitamin C, as well as carbohydrates in the form of natural sugars and fibre. To preserve the vitamin content, eat fruit raw and choose seasonal varieties since the highest concentration of vitamins is found in freshly picked fruit. Some dried fruits are a valuable source of iron but are also high in sugar and so should be eaten in moderation. Eat 5 or 6 portions per day from this group, if you can.

Olive oil, nuts, and seeds are good sources of monosaturated fats. The more expensive, cold-pressed oils, made without the use of heat or chemicals, are purer in content.

Dairy foods and dairy alternatives

Dairy products include whole milk, live natural yoghurt, cheese, butter, and cream. They provide a good source of complete protein, fats, calcium, and also the useful vitamin B12. Always choose dairy products which have been pasteurized. Organic dairy products are now widely available.

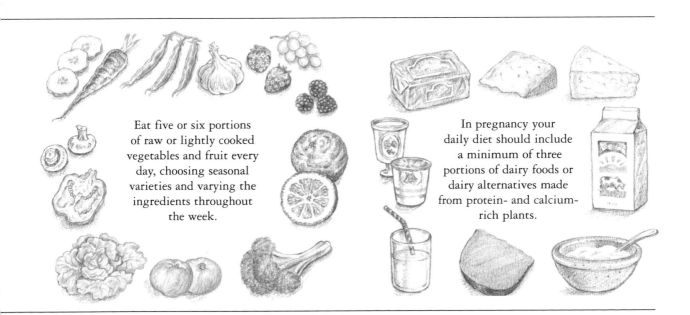

Eat five or six portions of raw or lightly cooked vegetables and fruit every day, choosing seasonal varieties and varying the ingredients throughout the week.

In pregnancy your daily diet should include a minimum of three portions of dairy foods or dairy alternatives made from protein- and calcium-rich plants.

Guidelines for vegetarians

Whether you eat a vegetarian or strictly vegan diet, you can follow much of the advice given on the previous pages. Dairy products, eggs, and honey may provide valuable sources of protein in a vegetarian diet, but if you are strictly vegan, excluding all animal products, you must make sure that you obtain sufficient vegetable protein from other sources, such as beans and nuts. Always include a choice from the cereal group in each meal, since this will aid the absorption of vegetable protein (see p. 25). Eat beans with rice or pasta, for example, or peanut butter with wholegrain bread. To ensure an adequate intake of protein while you are pregnant, include extra helpings of cereal foods and make sure that you eat protein from more than one source in each meal. Try to plan your weekly protein sources before shopping.

As a substitute for dairy foods, use organic soya milk and soya products. Mix calcium-rich sesame seed paste into salad dressings, sauces, or cakes, or add it to brown rice to give a lovely nutty taste.

Eat a wide variety of fresh vegetables and fruits each week; dried fruits, especially those containing iron (see p. 25), are useful but you should eat them in moderation since they have a high sugar content. Fresh-sprouted grains or beans are rich in nutrients (see p. 24) and can be eaten daily. You can use vitamin-B-rich yeast extract as a condiment or add it to sauces; brewer's yeast and molasses provide iron and other minerals. Include vitamin-C-rich foods in your daily diet to aid iron absorption and to increase your body's resistance to infection. If you are vegan, it is advisable to take a B12 vitamin supplement during pregnancy.

Seaweeds are a valuable source of proteins, minerals, and trace elements, particularly iodine, calcium, potassium, and iron, as well as some vitamins. Common types available include agar agar, carrageen, dulse, hizikmi, kombu, nori, and wakame. Add seaweed to your soups or sprinkle over your food. **Seaweeds have a high sodium content and should be avoided if you have high blood pressure.**

Nutritious drinks

Always drink according to your thirst in pregnancy, using bottled mineral or spring water rather than tap water. Avoid soft fizzy drinks/sodas, and instead of tea and coffee, drink mild herbal teas (see p. 63), and dandelion root or grain coffees. Alcohol is best avoided, although the occasional glass of wine will not harm you.

Fresh fruit and vegetable juices are highly nutritious and are best if you make them at home and drink them immediately. They are energizing and also have a cleansing and tonifying effect, but do not drink more than half a pint a day, since they are very concentrated. Apples, oranges, pears, beetroot/beets, carrots, celery, cucumber, lettuce, parsley, cabbage, spinach, and watercress are all suitable for juicing. Milk or yoghurt shakes are delicious and you can combine them with a variety of fruits.

Things to avoid

❖ Soft cheeses, unpasteurized dairy products and prepared salads have been associated with listeria poisoning. Do not eat in pregnancy or postnatally

❖ Refined and processed foods, particularly those with a high sugar or salt content, as well as very greasy or spicy foods

❖ Food additives, especially sodium nitrate and nitrite, and flavour enhancers, such as monosodium glutamate

❖ Intensively farmed meat, which may contain antibiotics

❖ Raw or rare meat and close contact with cat litter trays, since both are possible sources of the disease known as toxoplasmosis

❖ Stimulants such as tea and coffee, and cocoa and cola drinks, which all contain caffeine, as well as tranquillizers, aspirin, alcohol, and cigarettes

Healthy eating habits

The previous pages provide you with the broad guidelines for selecting a well-balanced and nutritious diet. It is important, however, to adjust the recommended quantities to suit your appetite, eating more, for example, if you are carrying twins or leading a very active life. You will, in any case, need to increase slightly the quantity of fats and carbohydrates in your diet while pregnant. If three substantial meals a day prove difficult to digest, try eating smaller amounts more frequently. Excessive weight gain (see p. 82) is unlikely if you are eating mainly wholefoods and plenty of fresh vegetables, fruit, and protein foods. Regular exercise (see pp. 30-43) will also help to ensure that your food is used effectively rather than stored as unnecessary weight.

If you long for sugary, refined foods then try to satisfy your craving with a more nutritious substitute. Nuts and raisins in moderate amounts or fresh vegetables make healthy, filling snacks between meals.

Use salt sparingly to taste but do not attempt to cut it out of your diet altogether. If possible, use pure sea salt from a health-food store. Organic soya sauce, tamari, and health-food vegetable stock powder contain small quantities of sea salt and may be used in moderation to flavour your foods.

When planning and preparing meals, take your time selecting foods and try to combine a variety of colours and textures both for added interest and to ensure a good mixture of nutrients. Lightly steam, stir fry, or bake fish and vegetables to retain maximum nutritional value. Try to create a comfortable, calm, and attractive setting in which to take your meals, preferably surrounded by plants and fresh air. Eat seated at a table and take your time, chewing your food well and remembering that the nourishment you are taking in is also going through to your baby.

CHAPTER 3

YOGA AND EXERCISE

Being at your physical best will help to ensure a healthy pregnancy and increase the possibility of a natural, active birth followed by a speedy recovery. In many indigenous societies, women live in harmony with nature, using their bodies in ways that promote suppleness, strength, and fitness. In so doing they naturally prepare themselves for birth and motherhood. Most of us, however, need to learn how to use our bodies as nature intended and exercising appropriately can make all the difference.

During the nine months of pregnancy, your body changes continually. Hormonal secretions relax and soften the ligaments that hold the joints together so that your skeleton becomes more flexible and expandable in preparation for birth. There is a general increase in body fluids, resulting in your heart having to work harder to ensure that the greater volume of blood is pumped throughout your body, and that an adequate supply reaches the placenta as well as your own vital organs. The workload of your kidneys is also heavier since they must filter and excrete waste products for both you and your baby. In addition, your digestion slows down due to hormonal softening of the muscles of the digestive tract.

The increase in suppleness that occurs means that your body responds more readily to yoga and exercise than at any other time, providing you with a unique opportunity for improving your flexibility. Practising the programme of basic yoga recommended on the following pages in combination with deep breathing (see p. 18) will improve all of your vital body functions, including circulation of fluids, elimination of waste, and respiration, as well as raising your general level of health and energy. Exercising regularly in this way will also help to prevent stress, release chronic tension, and protect your spine, so that your body can accommodate the changes of pregnancy with ease. As you gradually discover a greater degree of suppleness and freedom of movement, you will become increasingly comfortable in positions and movements that are natural to labour, at the same time as gaining confidence in your ability to cope with painful contractions. When the time comes to give birth you will know instinctively how to use your body, letting it flow with the contractions of your uterus as you allow yourself to let go.

Your daily exercise session will calm and centre you (see p. 18) and increase your awareness of your baby, bringing you stillness and inner peace so that you feel at one with yourself and your creative energy.

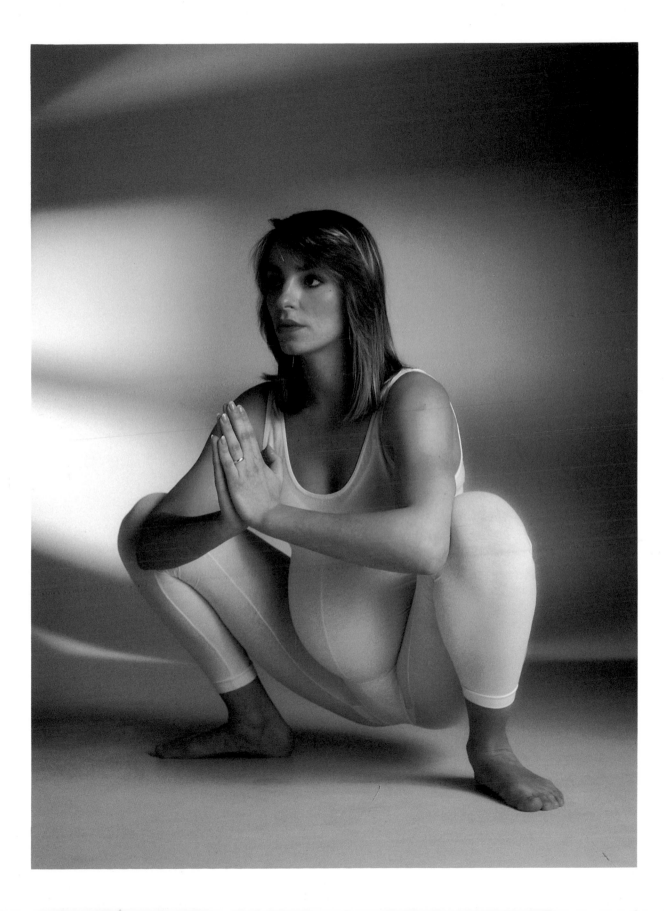

Daily exercise programme

The exercises described on the following pages are modified yoga positions. These are ideal for pregnancy since they are both gentle and non-strenuous. Some of the exercises are intended to strengthen specific muscle groups, while others encourage the softening and expansion of your pelvis to allow for the safe passage of your baby. When you practise yoga, your body finds a natural harmony with the Earth's energy. This is known as "grounding" and it is the key to a natural active birth, since it allows your body to relax in harmony with the downward pull of gravity so that you can release tension as you breathe. This is ideal preparation for the movements and spontaneous breathing that guide you through contractions in labour.

In addition to the programme of exercises, it is important to take regular, non-strenuous aerobic exercise, such as walking and swimming, which will stimulate your cardiovascular and respiratory systems. A walk in the open air each day will raise your energy level, encourage sound sleep, and help to position your baby correctly. Swimming daily or once or twice a week in a gentle and moderate way is highly beneficial. The Shaw method is ideal as it combines swimming with the Alexander Technique and is absolutely safe (see *The Art of Swimming,* p. 93). The buoyancy of the water gives you a sense of lightness and supports your weight so that you can exercise your body without strain. While it is important to practise yoga on land with the help of gravity, you may also enjoy experiementing with some positions in water.

Try to set aside an hour a day for breathing and exercise, choosing a time when you are unlikely to be interrupted. If you are not able to practise daily, then do so as often as you can. Find a suitable place to exercise with a free wall and a carpeted floor. If there is no carpet, use a couple of thick blankets instead. Create a pleasant setting by including plants, some attractive cushions, music, or anything else you find pleasurable.

A warm bath prior to exercising will help you to relax, especially first thing in the morning when your body may be a little stiff. Make sure you eat a light snack an hour or so before the session, but never exercise on a full stomach. Start with the deep breathing exercise described on page 18. Then begin exercising, taking your time and holding each position only for as long as it feels comfortable. At first you will probably be aware of the tightness in your body, but gradually you will learn how to release the tension through breathing, and your movements will come easier. If you feel like it, you can hold the positions for longer than indicated, but build up to this slowly. Always follow your exercise with a period of rest and relaxation (see p. 42).

Caution: While the exercises involving standing still, bending forward, and lying on the back are beneficial and enjoyable, a few women tend to feel lightheaded or dizzy due to the circulation changes that occur in these positions. Read the cautions carefully on these pages and leave out any exercises that affect you in this way. Should you feel faint at any time in your pregnancy, lie down on your left side and rest until you feel better; and, if you have some, take a few drops of the Bach Flower Rescue Remedy.

Stand with your feet about 30cm (12in) apart and parallel. Take a few deep breaths and, each time you exhale, imagine the breath travelling downward as your weight settles into your heels. Feel the outward breath pass through your heels into the ground, like the roots of a tree. Continue to breathe deeply and, starting with your feet, begin to work upward, becoming aware of each part of your body in turn.

Caution: Avoid this exercise if standing still makes you feel lightheaded or dizzy. Read it instead and use the suggestions when standing and walking normally.

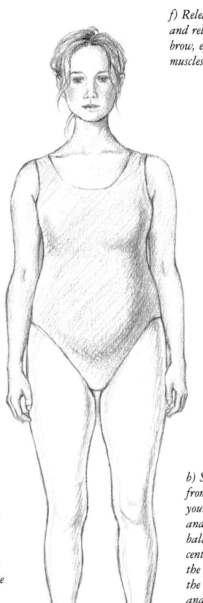

g) Drop your shoulders and allow your arms to hang comfortably down by your sides.

f) Release your jaw and relax your brow, eyes, and the muscles of your face.

e) Relax the back of your neck by dropping your chin down slightly toward your chest.

d) Gently release your lower back downward. This will bring your pelvis under your belly and prevent your back from arching.

c) Loosen your knees so that the energy can flow freely through your legs. Let your weight drop through your heels along with the downward pull of gravity.

a) Turn your heels out slightly wider than the toes, so that the outer edges of the feet are parallel. Lift and spread out your toes and then relax them so that your feet widen. Press down the base of your big toe and lift the inner arches of the feet. Finally, relax and feel your weight drop evenly into the floor through your heels.

b) Sway gently from your left to your right foot, and then find your balance in the centre. Be aware of the contact between the soles of your feet and the floor.

Postural awareness

During pregnancy, the extra weight of your growing baby and uterus alters the postural dynamics of your body so that the natural curves of your spine are exaggerated. Good posture ensures that the weight is transferred through your lower back to your hips, legs, and feet where it is discharged into the ground. Poor posture blocks the transfer of weight so that it accumulates, resulting in strain on the lower back, pelvis, and knees. Being mindful of your posture will reduce the possibility of backache and other skeletal pains as well as helping you to encourage your baby into a good position for birth.

When standing or walking, wear flat heeled shoes or sandals and try to keep your feet parallel; turning them out puts strain on the sacroiliac joints and can cause pain in the lower back and pelvis. Develop an awareness of the suggestions on page 33 and use them throughout your day. Avoid hollowing or arching your lower back when you stand or walk since this will tip your pelvis and the weight of your belly forward, placing strain on your lower back and abdominal muscles. Instead, gently lengthen your lower back downward so that your pelvis supports your abdomen evenly from underneath, and your baby is carried close to your spine as the weight is transferred to the ground.

Spend a minute or two standing like this and then walk a short distance in slow motion, bearing these suggestions in mind. With practice, you will notice how your posture finds its natural balance as your body moves forward gracefully in harmony with gravity.

When sitting at a desk or table, always try to keep your pelvis higher than your knees by placing a cushion or two on the seat of the chair and using another to support your back if necessary. Avoid slouching or semi-reclining with your feet up when watching television. In late pregnancy, this position may encourage your baby into a "posterior" lie with the baby's spine toward your spine and the limbs in front. This can sometimes, but not always, result in a longer labour with more back pain. Instead, sit upright with your lower back supported, or lie on your side, following the suggestions on page 42.

Lying frequently, but not always, on your left side encourages your baby into the most favourable "left anterior" position with the baby's spine on the left side of your abdomen. The following exercises will help you to develop postural awareness when sitting, kneeling, and lifting, and will also encourage your baby into an optimal position for birth.

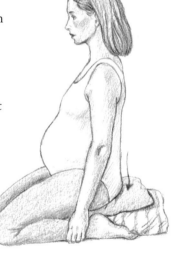

a) Kneel comfortably with your knees together and buttocks resting on a bolster or pile of three or four cushions, so that your pelvis is raised higher than your knees. Relax your lower back downward and let your weight drop through your hips.

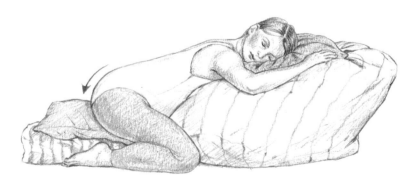

b) Still kneeling, spread your knees and slowly release your trunk forward, moving from your hips. Relax onto a beanbag or some large cushions, keeping your pelvis down. Both a) and b) release tension in the lower back and encourage optimal positioning of your baby.

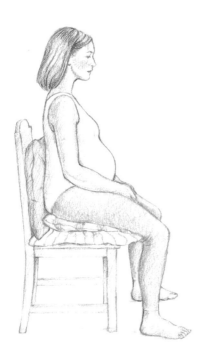

Sitting and squatting

In late pregnancy, sitting on a chair or squatting on a stool with your hips raised and your back vertical will reduce strain on your spine and encourage your baby's head to "engage" in the brim of the pelvis. Avoid slouching or semi-reclining at any time and don't do any deep squats (as on page 40) after 34 weeks.

c) Place two cushions on the seat of a chair and one behind your back, unless the chair has a straight back. Sit with your spine vertical and your lower back supported. Spread your legs apart and place your feet flat on the floor, heels down.

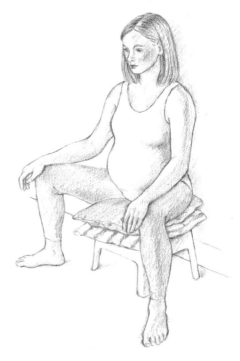

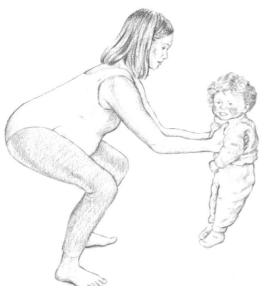

d) Put two or three cushions on a stool next to a wall. With feet comfortably wide apart and slightly turned out, lower yourself into a squat, positioning your lower back against the wall with your spine vertical.

e) To lift a toddler or heavy object, stand with your feet apart and slightly turned out, heels well grounded. Bend your knees into a semi-squat and lean forward from your hips, keeping your spine free. Drop your weight into your heels as you come up.

f) Kneel on your hands and knees and try gently swinging your hips from side to side, rotating or rocking forward and back. These movements in this position encourage your baby's spine to lie "anterior" in the curve of your belly, which is the best position for birth. They also release tension from your lower back.

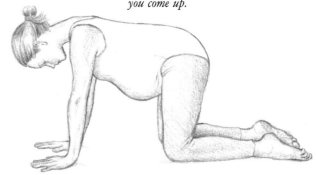

Tailor pose

This exercise improves circulation
in the pelvis and widens the
pelvic canal, increasing flexibility
of the joints and relaxing the
muscles of the pelvic floor. Sit on
the floor with your lower back
touching a wall. Bring the soles of
your feet together and place a
cushion under each knee. Relax
your arms, shoulders, and the
back of your neck.

*Breathe deeply, gently releasing your
lower back downward with the
exhalations so that your hips drop
softly toward the floor and your
weight centres in the pelvis. Then
gently lengthen your spine toward
the ceiling as you begin to inhale.
Continue like this for a minute or
two, and notice how tension releases
as you breathe.*

Sitting with legs wide apart

This exercise grounds the pelvis
and legs and releases tension in
the upper body. Sit on the floor
with your lower back touching a
wall. Spread your legs comfortably
wide apart and rest your hands on
your knees. Breathe deeply and let
your lower back, hips, pelvis, and
legs drop gently toward the floor
with each exhalation.

*As your lower body becomes more
grounded, feel a sense of lightness
and release moving up your spine
each time you begin to inhale. Relax
your neck and shoulders. Continue
like this for a minute or two, gently
extending your heels occasionally, to
bring the back of your knees closer to
the floor.*

Neck and shoulder release

Sit on the edge of a cushion and fold your legs so that one foot lies in front of the other, with a cushion under each knee. Relax and breathe deeply as you make these movements in sequence, releasing your lower back downward with the exhalations. Drop your pelvis, relax your arms and shoulders, and keep your spine vertical throughout.

a) Very slowly and smoothly, rotate your head three or four times in a soft circular movement. This releases tension in your neck. Bring your head back to the centre and repeat in the other direction.

b) Gently raise your arms above your head. Softly roll your elbows in and out a few times to release your shoulders, and then lower your arms. Repeat once or twice.

c) Raise one arm, bend the elbow, and place the palm in the centre of your upper back. Softly catch the elbow with your other hand, releasing your lower back downward. Hold for a few seconds, and repeat on the other side.

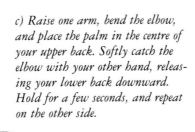

d) Turning gently to the right, hold behind your right knee with your left hand, and look over your right shoulder. Release your lower back downward, then return to the centre, and repeat on the left.

Pelvic release

This exercise releases tension in the groin, relaxes the muscles of the back and pelvic floor, and widens the pelvic outlet. It can be done with or without the help of a partner. Kneel with your knees apart, buttocks resting on your heels and your toes pointing inward. If this is uncomfortable, place a bolster lengthways between your legs or a couple of cushions under your hips.

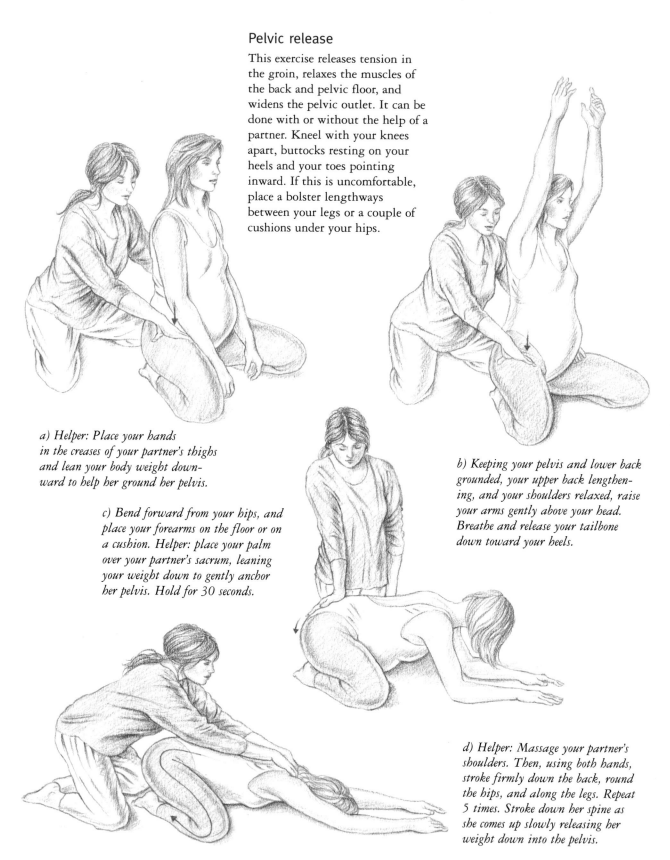

a) Helper: Place your hands in the creases of your partner's thighs and lean your body weight downward to help her ground her pelvis.

c) Bend forward from your hips, and place your forearms on the floor or on a cushion. Helper: place your palm over your partner's sacrum, leaning your weight down to gently anchor her pelvis. Hold for 30 seconds.

b) Keeping your pelvis and lower back grounded, your upper back lengthening, and your shoulders relaxed, raise your arms gently above your head. Breathe and release your tailbone down toward your heels.

d) Helper: Massage your partner's shoulders. Then, using both hands, stroke firmly down the back, round the hips, and along the legs. Repeat 5 times. Stroke down her spine as she comes up slowly releasing her weight down into the pelvis.

Shoulder stretch

This exercise relaxes the chest and shoulders, and improves breathing. It may also relieve heartburn and will tone the muscles that support the breasts. Position yourself facing a wall with your knees wide apart and your pelvis on your heels. Gently raise your arms and place your hands about 30cm (12in) apart on the wall.

Drop your shoulders, keeping your elbows straight and your hands as high as possible, and release your lower back down toward your heels. Breathe deeply and hold for a few seconds. Come up and roll your shoulders. Repeat a few times.

Forward bend

This exercise relaxes the muscles of the pelvic floor and those at the back of the legs. Stand with your feet 30cm (12in) apart and parallel and your hands linked behind you.

Caution: Avoid leaning forward if it makes you feel dizzy or lightheaded.

Pelvic tuck-in

This exercise reduces stress on the lower back. Kneel on all fours with your knees and your palms about 30cm (12in) apart. Relax your neck and breathe deeply.

a) Lengthen your lower back and tuck your pelvis under so that your spine arches and your tailbone points down toward your heels. Hold for a few seconds, then release. Repeat 5 to 10 times. To relieve backache, repeat several times a day.

Dropping your heels, slowly bend forward from the hips, keeping your trunk long and your neck relaxed. Breathe deeply. Hold for a few cycles of breath, then come up slowly.

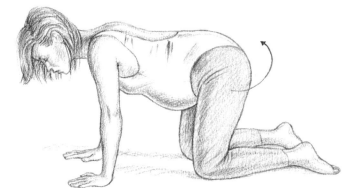

b) Breathing deeply, roll your pelvis clockwise in big, wide circles, focusing on long, slow exhalations. Repeat in the other direction. These movements may also be useful for coping with strong contractions in labour.

Squatting

Squatting opens your pelvis and is an effective position for birth. Stand with your feet 45cm (18in) apart. Turn them out slightly and bend your knees as you lower your pelvis into a squat. Keep your heels down if you can.

a) Keep your heels down or rock from one foot to the other. Spread your knees apart with your elbows. If necessary, use a wall to support your back or squat on a low stool.

Caution: Avoid deep squats like these in the last six weeks of pregnancy (see alternative on p. 35).

b) Alternatively, stand, holding each other's wrists, with elbows straight and heels down. Lower yourself into a squat. Hold for a few seconds, then come up. Repeat 3 times. Helper: place one foot in front of the other. Lean back to avoid straining.

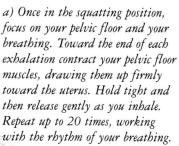

a) Once in the squatting position, focus on your pelvic floor and your breathing. Toward the end of each exhalation contract your pelvic floor muscles, drawing them up firmly toward the uterus. Hold tight and then release gently as you inhale. Repeat up to 20 times, working with the rhythm of your breathing.

b) Use the knee-chest position for the pelvic floor exercise described under a) if you have a cervical stitch (see p. 91), varicosities (see p. 79), or if your baby is breech (see p. 90) after 34 weeks. This position can also help to slow down intense contractions in labour.

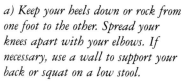

Pelvic floor exercise

This exercise relaxes and strengthens the muscles of the pelvic floor and helps to prevent prolapse. Either adopt position **a)**, squatting on your toes with your hands on the floor. Or use position **b)**, kneeling with your head on your arms.

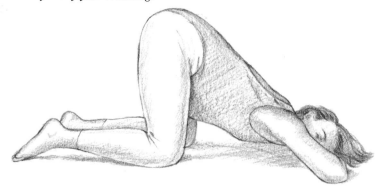

Caution: The exercises on this page involve lying on your back and may be done throughout pregnancy up to 34 weeks. In the last six weeks, or if you feel uncomfortable or dizzy when lying on your back, then leave out these positions. To come out of the position, roll onto one side, rest there for a moment and then come up slowly.

Inner thigh stretch

This exercise releases tension in the inner thigh muscles and improves venous return. Sit down sideways with one hip touching the wall. Swing round and lie down in one movement, bringing your legs up against the wall at a right angle to your body. Make sure your buttocks are touching the wall and your upper body is straight. Getting into this position will become easier after a little practice.

a) Breathe deeply into your belly and release your spine, bringing the back of your waist down onto the floor. Tuck your chin in and lengthen the back of your neck. Relax your shoulders, jaw, and face. Extend your heels.

b) Breathe out and spread your legs, gently extending your heels. Release your lower back toward the floor and softly take your arms over your head and place them on the floor. Relax and breathe, bending your knees as in squatting to take a rest. Continue for one or two minutes.

c) Bend your knees and bring the soles of your feet together as close to your body as possible. Press your knees gently toward the wall using your hands. Hold for 30 seconds and then slowly roll onto your side to come up.

Relaxation

It is important to follow your daily exercise session with 10 to 30 minutes of rest and relaxation. Choose one of the comfortable positions illustrated, using plenty of cushions so that your body is well supported. Concentrate your awareness on the rhythm of your breathing, allowing your body to sink deeper and deeper into relaxation with each exhalation. Starting with your toes, feet, and ankles, work gradually up through your calves and thighs toward your pelvis. Breathe into the pelvic area and the pelvic floor and feel the whole area soften and relax as you exhale. Be aware of the gentle curves of your spine and release your upper back and shoulders. Take the breath through to your arms, hands, palms, and fingertips, and then exhale and release. Relax your neck, throat, and the corners of your jaw, and release all the tiny muscles of the face so that your brow becomes completely smooth. Let your eyes sink deep into their sockets and feel your eyelids lengthen and soften. Be aware of the breath as it enters your nostrils and, still concentrating on the gentle wave of the breath, sink deeper and deeper into relaxation. Once you are totally relaxed and comfortable, bring your attention to the presence of the baby you are carrying inside you and spend some quiet moments resting and relaxing in peace together (see p. 21). At the end of the resting period, refresh yourself with a drink of herbal tea or fruit juice.

Resting positions

Use the following positions to rest and relax after exercising. After 34 weeks avoid using position b), and kneel forward over cushions (see opposite) as an alternative resting position.

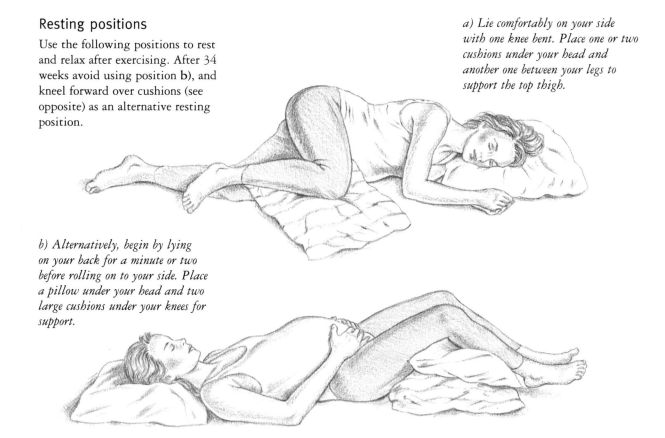

a) Lie comfortably on your side with one knee bent. Place one or two cushions under your head and another one between your legs to support the top thigh.

b) Alternatively, begin by lying on your back for a minute or two before rolling on to your side. Place a pillow under your head and two large cushions under your knees for support.

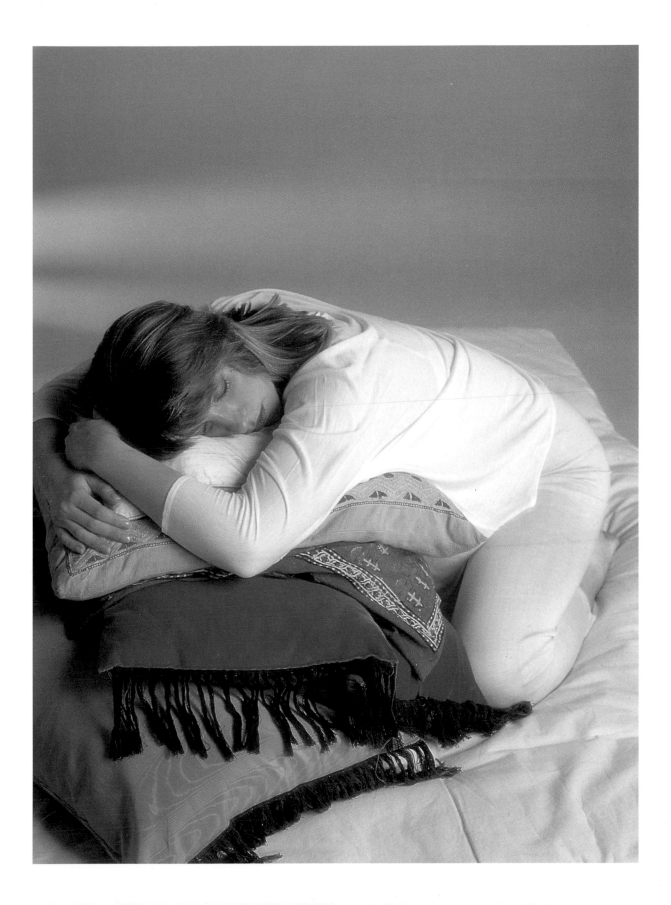

CHAPTER 4

MASSAGE

Throughout life, we communicate, show affection, and comfort one another by touching. Our sensitivity to touch develops early while we are still in the womb. Stimulation of the nerve endings in the skin by the surrounding amniotic fluid gives us our first awareness of the boundaries of self. From birth through to old age, touch in the form of massage can be used for healing and relaxation, to awaken the senses and quieten the mind, and to bring us back into harmony with ourselves.

In some countries, such as India and Japan, massage is an essential part of the midwife's skill and as such is used to prepare both mother and baby for birth and the postnatal period. Many women also find massage effective as a means of relieving pain in labour. It is said to stimulate the release of hormones, known as endorphins, which act as natural relaxants, pain-killers, and euphorics during both pregnancy and birth.

Regular massage will help to balance your energies and prevent ill health. Physiologically, it stimulates and regulates the body, improving the flow of blood and lymph so that oxygen, nutrients, and waste products are carried more effectively to and from your own body tissues and the placenta. By relieving tension and encouraging the release of pent-up emotions, massage relaxes and soothes the nerves and may also help to lower blood pressure. If you are unwell, it will enhance your body's own healing potential and in this way can be used to complement the natural therapies described in Chapter 5.

Perhaps most important of all, massage nourishes you, making you feel valued and cared for. It is a way of sharing energy that benefits both giver and receiver. The sequences illustrated on pages 48-54 focus on ways in which your partner can massage you during pregnancy, but you may enjoy reciprocating and can either adapt the sequences intuitively or enhance your skills by further reading (see p. 93).

Massage can be an exquisitely sensual experience, inducing a state of meditative tranquillity in both giver and receiver that is perfect preparation for birth. It puts you in touch with your partner and, during the latter months of pregnancy, your unborn child may also be aware of your belly being gently stroked and caressed. Regular shared massage as well as self-massage will help you to trust your body and to relax and open up to the natural processes that take over when you give birth. It will also teach you how to use massage to soothe and calm your baby during infancy.

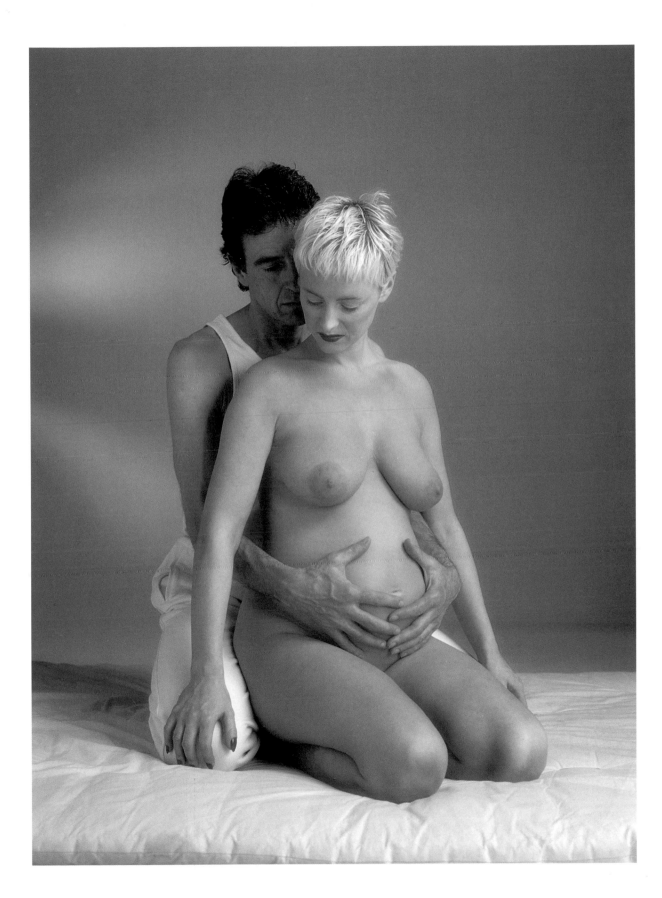

Self-massage

Massaging yourself daily after bathing, using a stretchmark prevention oil (see p. 77), will help to maintain elasticity of the skin during pregnancy. While there is no way of guaranteeing that you won't get stretchmarks, massaging and nourishing your skin will certainly help to prevent them. The areas to concentrate on are the belly, hips, thighs, and breasts, but other parts of the body, such as face, feet, and calves, are also easy to massage by yourself.

Breast massage

Breast massage helps to lubricate and soften the skin around the nipples and areolae. The milk-producing cells are arranged in little clusters in your breasts, rather like miniature bunches of grapes. When you feed your baby, the milk is ejected from these cells into ducts that run toward the nipples. When massaging, use a pure almond oil and work your way round each breast, stroking from the circumference to the nipple in the direction of the ducts. You may find it helpful to think of the face of a clock and to work gradually clockwise starting at the figure one. Massage with your whole hand, keeping your fingers together. Use a smooth even pressure, starting each stroke with the heel of the palm and continuing through to the fingers.

Your breasts produce their own lubricating fluid during pregnancy and you may notice the oil glands around the areolae becoming more pronounced. Avoid using soap on your breasts when washing since this tends to remove

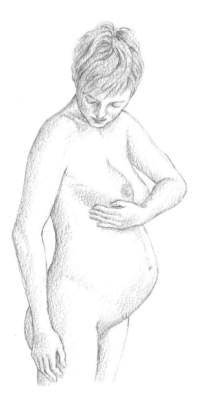

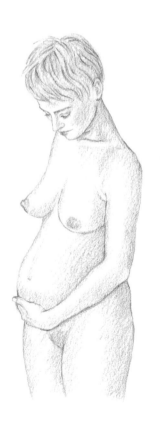

Pregnancy breast massage

Using the palm and fingers of one hand, massage in a clockwise direction around the whole of the breast, stroking from the circumference toward the nipple. Use almond oil or calendula cream and stroke firmly but gently with an even pressure. Massage the nipple with your fingers and thumb.

Belly massage

Pour plenty of oil into the hand, rub your palms together, and then apply the oil to your belly with smooth circular strokes, working in a clockwise direction. Be aware of your baby inside as you massage your belly. In the later months, he or she will probably be able to feel your touch. Continue to oil and massage your hips and thighs and the rest of your body.

the natural oils. Toward the end of your pregnancy, you may notice a few drops of the yellowish fluid known as colostrum coming from the openings in your nipples. This is the wonderfully nutritious "first milk" that your body produces for your baby in the first day or two after birth, and it is quite normal for it to appear during pregnancy.

Breast care

Your breasts do not require preparation for feeding during pregnancy. Your midwife or doctor will examine them once in early pregnancy to check that the nipples are not inverted (see p. 76). It is advisable to wear a supportive bra, preferably one with a high cotton content, throughout your pregnancy. Make sure you are properly fitted by an expert to allow room for growth. There is no need to wear a bra at night and it is a good idea to go without one sometimes during the day. It is also agreeable to expose your breasts to mild sunshine or open air from time to time. Three weeks before your due date is a good time to be fitted for the special nursing bras that you will need after the birth (see *Useful Addresses*, p. 93 for bra suppliers).

Belly massage

It is best to begin massaging your belly daily from early pregnancy onward. To increase elasticity and tone the skin, use a pure wheatgerm or almond oil as a base oil (see recipe below). When massaging, use plenty of oil and work with your whole hand or both hands at once. You will enjoy feeling your belly's lovely rounded shape and as pregnancy advances you will become increasingly aware of your baby's presence inside you. Continue working down your hips and thighs, using both hands to massage and oiling thoroughly with smooth, circular strokes.

Toward the end of your pregnancy, massage down the sides of your belly, from the ribs toward the navel, to prevent stress and to improve the elasticity of your abdominal muscles.

Perineal massage

In the last weeks of pregnancy, you can help to prepare yourself for birth by massaging the perineal tissues (the fleshy area between the vagina and anus) with almond, olive, or wheatgerm oil after bathing. This is easiest done in a half-kneeling position with one leg up, or a squatting position (see p. 35) using the thumb and fingers of one hand. Your partner may also be willing to help. Massage softens and increases the stretchability of the perineal tissues prior to birth and can help to prevent tearing.

Belly oil

50ml (1¾ fl oz) of wheatgerm or almond oil
essential oils of neroli and sweet orange

Add 5 drops of each essential oil to your choice of base oil. Use this oil to massage your belly in pregnancy but avoid using essential oils on your breasts when you are breastfeeding.

Daily massage by a partner

While there are many different types of massage, this chapter focuses on a simple intuitive style of massage that is easy to learn and suitable for use in pregnancy. The emphasis is on self-discovery and you will find that, with a little practice, your own natural skills will emerge. The massage strokes recommended fall into three groups – light stroking over the surface, kneading muscles (rather like kneading dough), and applying firm but gentle pressure, which goes a little deeper. Soon you will begin to improvise on the basic strokes and develop your own individual style.

You will need a warm, quiet place in which to massage, some comfortable cushions, and a bottle of aromatic oil (see *Aromatherapy,* p. 66), either made up from one of the recipes given below or bought ready prepared (see p. 93 for suppliers of preblended aromatherapy oils for use in pregnancy). It is also a good idea to have a warm towel to place over parts of the body that are not being massaged. Slow-burning incense may help to enhance the experience.

Whether you are giving or receiving massage, it is important to be relaxed and comfortable. Allow a little time to centre yourself beforehand, using the deep-breathing exercise on page 18. During the massage it is best for both of you to focus on your breathing and to avoid talking more than necessary.

Giving a massage

Before you start to massage, take some time to tune in to your partner's energy, and that of the baby she is carrying inside her, by touching her body lightly with both hands. Then warm some oil in your hands by rubbing your palms together, and apply lightly to the part of the body you are about to massage. Spread the oil evenly over the whole area. Then sit or kneel comfortably beside your partner and breathe deeply to relax and centre yourself. Begin to work, starting slowly and keeping your mind on the sensations you are feeling. Try to put your whole body into the movements and make sure you are fully relaxed. Ask your partner how she is feeling and take time to discover the delights of this health-giving practice together.

Refreshing pregnancy body oil

50ml (1¾ fl oz) of grapeseed or almond oil
essential oils of lemon, grapefruit, and sweet orange

Add 5 drops of each of the essential oils to your choice of base oil. This massage oil has a fresh citrus smell and can be used as an alternative to stretchmark prevention oil (see p. 77) after bathing.

Euphoric and relaxing pregnancy oil

50ml (1¾ fl oz) of grapeseed or almond oil
essential oils of bergamot and ylang ylang

Add 5 drops of each of the essential oils to your choice of base oil. This massage oil is uplifting and will help to alleviate depression.

Upper and lower back massage

Ask your partner to kneel and lean forward over a pile of cushions so that her whole body is comfortably supported. Encourage her to breathe deeply and relax. Place your hands lightly on her body and, breathing deeply yourself, tune into her energy.

a) Oil your hands and place them on your partner's shoulders. Using your palms, fingers, and thumbs, knead the shoulder muscles, the back of the neck, and the upper back, increasing the pressure as needed.

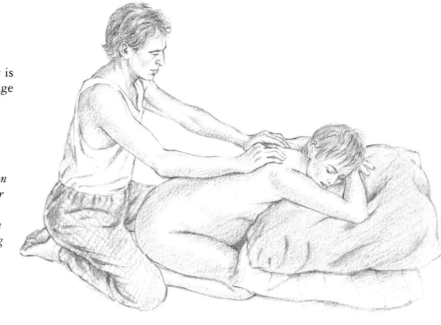

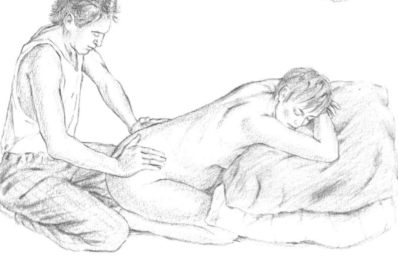

b) Massage down the spine from the neck to the lower back, pausing to work on any tight or tender spots. Use the heel of your palms and also your thumbs and fingers to massage the lower back. Start with the triangular sacral bone and work from the centre outward, covering the hips, buttocks, and thighs.

Neck and arm massage

Ask your partner to kneel, and position yourself so that you are kneeling comfortably behind her.

Using the fingers of both hands, work into the muscles of your partner's neck and shoulders. Then knead the shoulders firmly, using the whole of each hand. Work down the upper arms, squeezing and releasing the muscles. Massage each lower arm and hand separately.

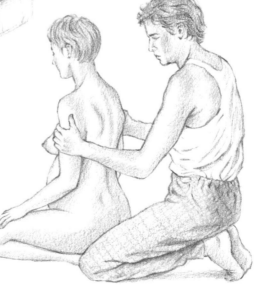

Face massage

Ask your partner to sit down
with her upper body well
supported by cushions and higher
than her legs. Place some additional cushions under her knees.
Kneel or sit comfortably behind
her and take her head gently
between your hands so that the
tips of your fingers are resting at
the base of her skull.

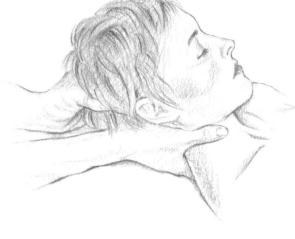

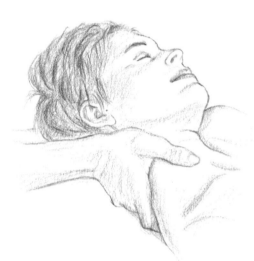

*a) Encourage your partner to breathe
deeply and let go so that her head
relaxes in your hands. Massage up
the back of her neck with long, even
strokes. Then, supporting her neck
with one hand, massage the back of
the skull with the other.*

*b) Roll your partner's head gently to
one side. Massage with the heel of
your palm down the side of her neck.
Repeat on the other side.*

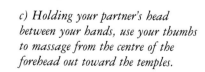

*c) Holding your partner's head
between your hands, use your thumbs
to massage from the centre of the
forehead out toward the temples.*

*d) Massage along the upper rims of
the eye sockets, working out from the
centre. Next massage the lower rims
of the eye sockets, again working
outward.*

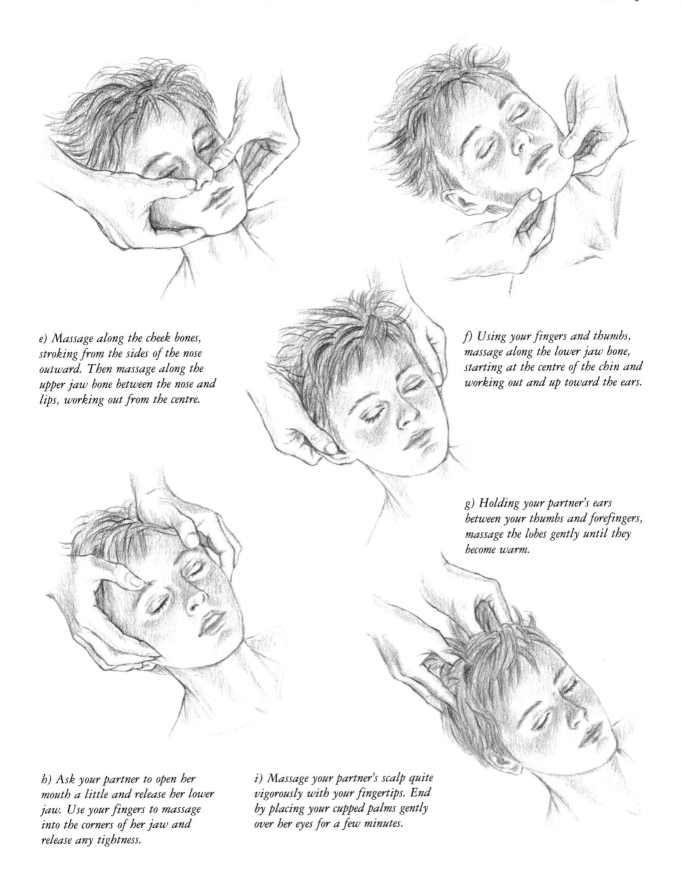

e) Massage along the cheek bones, stroking from the sides of the nose outward. Then massage along the upper jaw bone between the nose and lips, working out from the centre.

f) Using your fingers and thumbs, massage along the lower jaw bone, starting at the centre of the chin and working out and up toward the ears.

g) Holding your partner's ears between your thumbs and forefingers, massage the lobes gently until they become warm.

h) Ask your partner to open her mouth a little and release her lower jaw. Use your fingers to massage into the corners of her jaw and release any tightness.

i) Massage your partner's scalp quite vigorously with your fingertips. End by placing your cupped palms gently over her eyes for a few minutes.

Whole body massage

The following massage sequence will encourage total relaxation and help to ensure restful sleep. Breathing deeply, take your time and work slowly.

a) Ask your partner to lie on her side and kneel comfortably behind her. Use your thumbs to massage the long muscles that run down either side of her spine. Start from the top of her neck and work down to her pelvis, loosening any tight spots with small, circular movements.

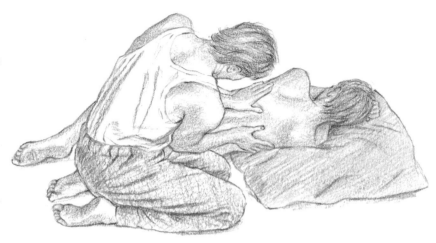

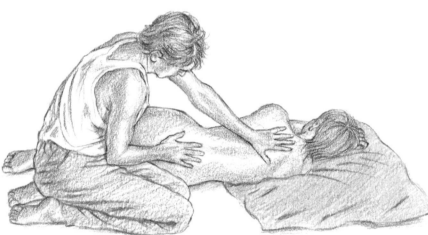

b) Using the palm of one hand, start at the base of your partner's neck and massage down the length of her spine with long, even strokes. Alternate your hands to create a regular, soothing rhythm.

c) Using one hand, massage around the hip bone and buttock muscles, working into any stiff or painful areas with your thumb. Ask your partner to turn over and repeat on her other side.

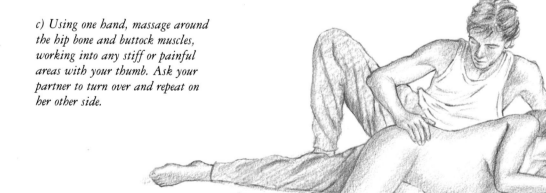

d) Use plenty of oil to massage your partner's belly. Spread the oil over the centre of her belly and then massage around the side, making circular strokes in a clockwise direction. Work with your whole hand, using a light, even pressure.

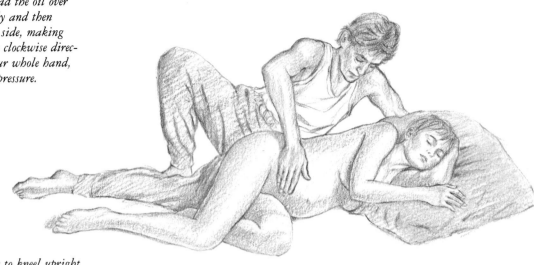

e) Ask your partner to kneel upright and position yourself close behind so that you are cradling both mother and baby in your arms. Breathing deeply, encourage your partner to do the same and to focus with you on the presence of her baby. Begin to stroke her belly gently, sensing the baby's movements with your hands.

f) Ask your partner to stand with her feet slightly apart and parallel. Working on one leg at a time, place your hands to either side of your partner's calf and massage upward with circular strokes. Continue massaging in the same way up her thigh. Then massage down the centre of the back of her leg, using your thumbs and working from the buttock down to the heel. Repeat on the other leg.

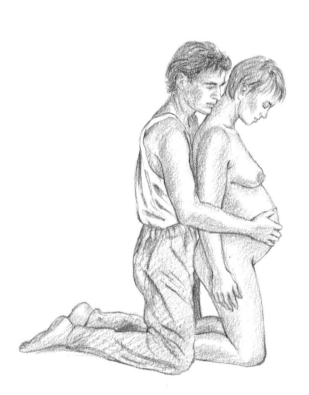

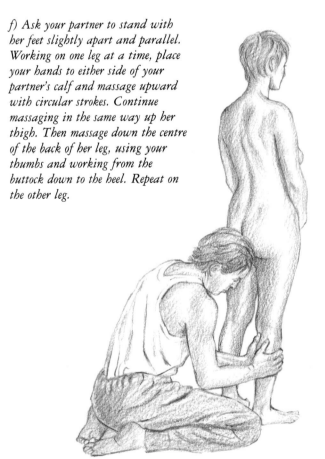

Foot massage

Encourage your partner to
recline comfortably against a
pile of cushions. Take her heel in
one hand and support her lower
leg on your knee.

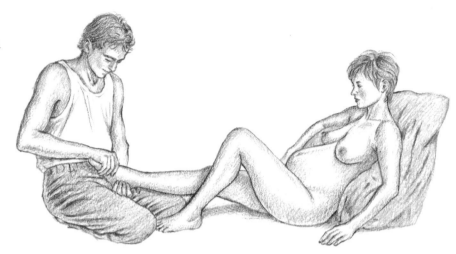

Caution: In pregnancy, avoid
massage of the heel, ankle
bones, and achilles tendon.
Reflexologists consider these
parts of the foot to be related
to the uterus and deep massage
may stimulate contractions.
During labour, however,
massage of these areas may
help to relieve pain.

*a) Using your free hand, stroke
from the top to the bottom of your
partner's foot. Continue to work
intuitively over the whole foot,
bending, flexing, and rotating it
in your hands.*

*b) Using the heel of your hand, press
up into the arch of your partner's foot.
Work back toward the heel and apply
firm, rhythmic pressure. This will
help to relieve tension in the arch.*

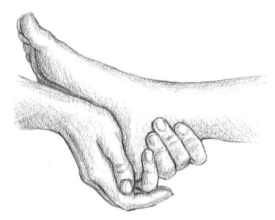

*c) Using both thumbs, massage the
sole of your partner's foot. Then,
supporting the arch with one hand,
grasp hold of her toes with the other
and flex them up and down. Repeat
5 times.*

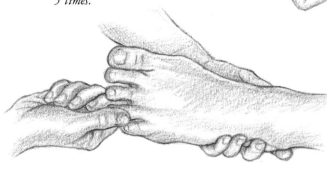

*d) Supporting your partner's foot in
one hand, use the other hand to
work each toe individually. Bend
the toe back and forward, then
stroke up and down each side. Next
rotate the toe slowly, three times in
each direction. Finally, pull the toe
toward you.*

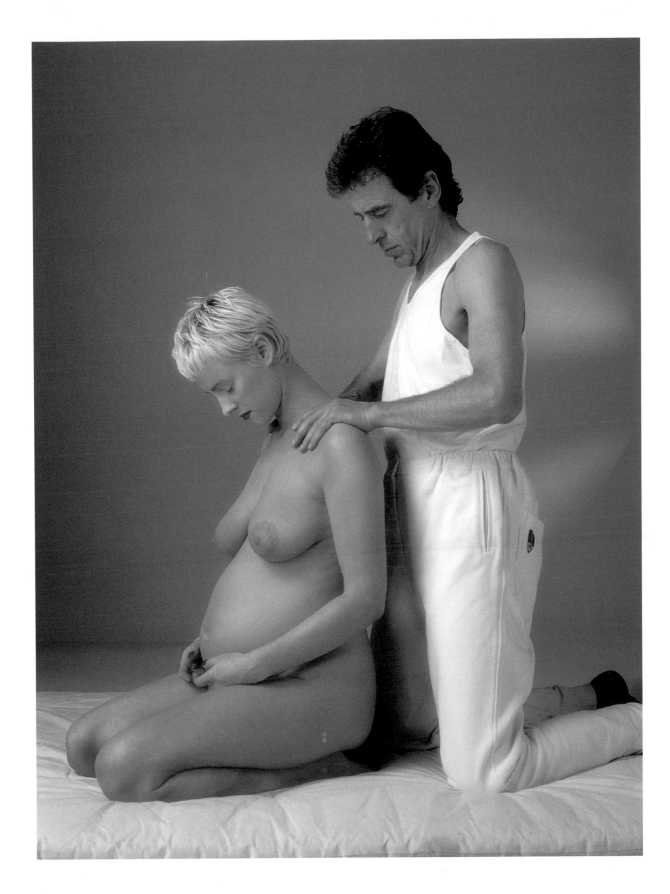

CHAPTER 5

NATURAL THERAPIES

All of us have the potential for self-healing and natural therapies work to enhance and strengthen this ability. Collectively referred to as complementary or alternative medicine, they follow a holistic approach, treating the whole person rather than just the symptoms manifesting at a particular time. When an ailment occurs during pregnancy, a holistic practitioner will consider all aspects of the problem, including the underlying causes. Treatment will aim both to correct any malfunction of energy and to raise your general level of health, thereby strengthening your natural defences. When used appropriately, natural therapies have no dangerous or unpleasant side effects and are safe for use in pregnancy. They provide a viable alternative to drug therapy and surgery which are generally not recommended at this time.

The therapies described in the following pages are effective in treating many of the ailments that are common in pregnancy (see pp. 69-92). You may also use them when you are in good health in order to maintain vital energy and optimal wellbeing in the months approaching birth. People respond differently to the various therapies and you will probably find that some are more useful to you than others.

All natural therapies aim to reach the subtle energies of the body, although the means by which they do so may vary significantly. Osteopathy and acupuncture, for example, are applied to the outside of the body, while herbalism and homeopathy involve ingestion of natural remedies derived from the environment. With the guidance of a practitioner, you can combine some therapies effectively, but others may be incompatible. Herbalism, for example, may work well with acupuncture, whereas aromatherapy and homeopathy are not always complementary since some essential oils can counteract the effects of certain homeopathic remedies.

In using the word "natural", it is important not to underestimate the powerful effects that these therapies can have. In pregnancy especially, it is wise to consult a skilled practitioner for initial guidance, and preferably one who has experience of working with pregnant women. Enquire at the outset about the likely cost of your treatment, which may vary from reasonable to expensive depending on the individual practitioner and the number of sessions you are likely to require. Sometimes treatment can continue in the form of self-help at home; in other instances regular consultation may be necessary.

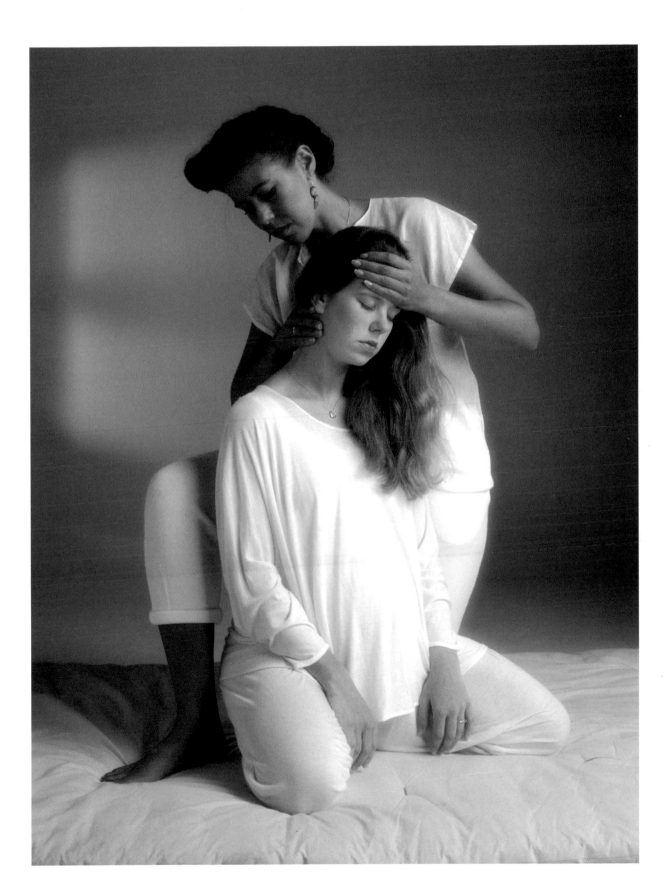

Osteopathy

Osteopathy is based on the belief that our skeletal framework and organ systems are interdependent. Consequently, the body will only function at its best and utilize its full self-healing potential if the structure is correctly aligned so that the muscles can work harmoniously in relation to gravity and the fluids are able to circulate freely.

By correcting structural imbalances in the spine and other areas, osteopathy improves blood flow to the organs and nerves, and thus has a beneficial effect on the whole body. It is particularly helpful in pregnancy when your posture changes as a result of the softening of the ligaments that bind your joints. As your body adjusts to your altered posture and the weight of the growing baby, unusual aches and pains can occur (see pp. 83-84) and underlying structural problems may be highlighted. A skilled practitioner who is used to treating pregnant women will work gently, manipulating and stretching tissues, to assist the body to accommodate the dynamic changes and to cope with the additional weight. Areas most commonly stressed are the neck, head, lower back, pelvic joints, and front pubic joint, but you may also feel pain in the upper spine, shoulders, ribs, wrists, knees, and feet. During pregnancy, treatment is often most effective if given regularly, since the body is constantly changing.

Cranial osteopathy is based on the discovery that the bones of the skull move and can be gently manipulated by a trained practitioner. It is a subtle and yet powerful form of treatment, believed to have a positive effect on the circulation of the cerebrospinal fluid that bathes the entire nervous system. It may be used to influence all parts of the body and can relieve the structural pains mentioned above. It is also helpful for depression, insomnia, and physical and psychological trauma. Cranial osteopathy works well in pregnancy when your body is at its most responsive and structural irregularities are easiest to put right. Your newborn baby may also benefit from treatment if birth was in any way traumatic.

What to expect

At your first osteopathy session, a detailed case history will be taken and a series of questions may be put to you about the nature and origin of your complaint. You will then be asked to remove your outer garments and to sit, stand, and lie down so that the therapist can observe the way you use your body. The actual treatment lasts about half an hour and usually takes place while you are lying or sitting on an osteopathic couch. The osteopath may use a combination of stretching movements, manipulation, and pressure to relax tense body tissues and muscles, and may also take the affected joint through its normal range of movements to restore mobility. You may be given exercises to practise at home as well as nutritional advice. Any aching following treatment will soon pass but you should arrange to rest after each session.

A cranial osteopath works mainly on the head and sacrum. While cranial manipulation is almost imperceptible at the time, you may experience a sudden release of energy or a profound need to sleep or rest later on.

Reflexology

Reflexology works on the premise that there are areas on the feet and hands (see below) that reflect different parts of the body. If an area feels sensitive or painful to the touch, the organ to which it is connected may be weak; therapeutic massage of the foot or hand is then used to heal and strengthen the affected organ. Reflexology is an effective treatment for many minor ailments, including stress, headaches, digestive problems, migraine, and sinusitis. It is essential during pregnancy, however, to seek professional advice before attempting to treat yourself.

What to expect

A trained reflexologist will use your feet or hands for both diagnosis and treatment. The therapist identifies sensitive areas by bending and releasing his or her thumb, for example, so that it works its way across the base of your foot. He or she then uses pressure and gentle thumb massage to promote healing. The beneficial effects of reflexology can be remarkable, although you may experience some mild pain during treatment.

Caution: Use only gentle pressure during pregnancy and avoid the heels, ankles, and achilles tendon, since these areas are connected to the uterus and massage may stimulate contractions.

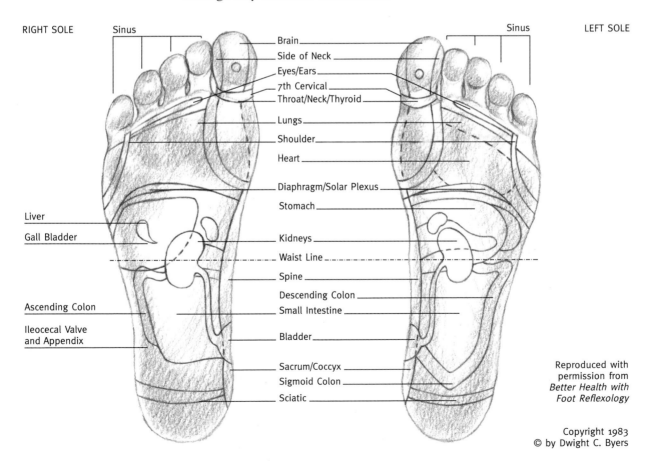

RIGHT SOLE · Sinus · Sinus · LEFT SOLE

Brain
Side of Neck
Eyes/Ears
7th Cervical
Throat/Neck/Thyroid
Lungs
Shoulder
Heart
Diaphragm/Solar Plexus
Stomach
Kidneys
Waist Line
Spine
Descending Colon
Small Intestine
Bladder
Sacrum/Coccyx
Sigmoid Colon
Sciatic

Liver
Gall Bladder
Ascending Colon
Ileocecal Valve and Appendix

Reproduced with permission from *Better Health with Foot Reflexology*

Copyright 1983 © by Dwight C. Byers

Acupuncture

Acupuncture originated in China over 5000 years ago and is now widely practised in the West. It is based on the concept of there being a vital life force or flow of energy in the body, known as "chi". This energy is both a manifestation of the universal life force around us and the animating principle that makes life possible.

Within our bodies, the chi flows through channels, or "meridians" (see opposite), which are linked to different organs. In order to experience health and harmony, the energy must flow freely. An acupuncturist uses very fine needles to release blockages and to stimulate points along the meridians, thus correcting imbalances and restoring equilibrium.

Acupuncture is practised only by trained professionals. It is effective in treating a wide range of functional disorders, including bladder and kidney problems, aches and pains, high blood pressure, digestive disorders, skin problems, and tiredness. It can also be used to stimulate labour and to turn babies who are in the breech position. Regular sessions will help you to maintain health and energy throughout your pregnancy.

What to expect

At the start of an acupuncture session, the practitioner will want to know details of your medical history and may ask you questions relating to your lifestyle and general wellbeing. He or she will observe your appearance and check for imbalances of energy by feeling your wrist pulse. You will then be asked to remove your outer garments and lie down. During pregnancy, it is advisable to lie on your side or sit up during treatment, or else lie on your back with a large cushion under your knees (see p. 42).

You will be encouraged to relax and breathe deeply while the therapist inserts a few very fine needles into specific points along the meridians. This is a virtually painless process, since the needles usually penetrate only the superficial skin layers. Don't be surprised, however, if they are inserted into an area of your body where you are not experiencing symptoms, since any of the points along a given meridian may be stimulated to influence the relevant organ. Once the needles have been inserted, you are unlikely to feel more than a mild tingling sensation, but as the energy flow improves you should experience a growing sense of wellbeing. The needles may be removed after a minute or two or left in for up to 30 minutes. No pain is felt on removal.

The therapist may employ different techniques to stimulate points, including finger pressure (see *Shiatsu,* p. 62), massage, and moxibustion, a form of heat treatment that uses a bundle of dried leaves of a slow-burning, pungent herb, known as moxa. The end is lit and held a short distance from the skin for a few seconds at a time so that the heat penetrates the point without burning the skin. Moxa may also be laid briefly on the skin so that it heats but does not burn the surface area, or it may be applied to the end of a needle.

Caution: Certain points should not be used in pregnancy, so it is important to consult a practitioner who works regularly with pregnant women.

There are twelve pairs of energy channels, or meridians, in the body. Two additional channels run down the front and back midlines and six extra meridians link the whole system. Energy, or chi, flows through this network of meridians, animating every part of the body. The spleen, stomach, and kidney meridians (coloured in brown) are those that nourish the uterus, placenta, and baby during pregnancy and birth.

a) Large intestine
b) Lung
c) Spleen
d) Stomach
e) Kidney
f) Midline
g) Liver
h) Gall Bladder

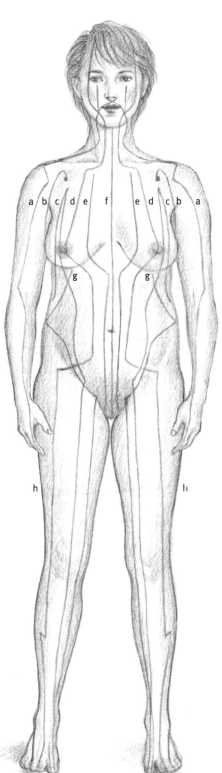

Shiatsu

Shiatsu evolved from *amna*, the traditional form of Japanese massage, and involves the use of finger pressure rather than needles to stimulate acupuncture points along the meridians. Basic shiatsu techniques are effective as self-help remedies for many common ailments in pregnancy, but you will need to consult a practitioner for a full treatment.

What to expect

On a first visit, a thorough case history will be taken and you will be asked to lie down comfortably on the floor wearing only light clothing. When pregnant, you may feel most comfortable in one of the positions recommended in Chapter 4. The therapist will gently but firmly apply pressure, or "shiatsu", with fingers, thumbs, palms, and sometimes knees and elbows, using body-weight rather than force.

Where basic shiatsu is recommended as a self-help remedy for a particular ailment in Chapter 6, follow the specific instructions given.

Caution: Shiatsu should not be used on the abdomen during pregnancy nor should direct pressure be applied to varicose veins. In late pregnancy, avoid heavy pressure on the legs.

Herbalism

Herbalism uses plants, drawn from a wide spectrum of fruit and vegetable species, for their cleansing and healing properties and is perhaps the oldest natural therapy we know. Herbs take up substances that your body needs from the earth and can benefit your health generally, stimulating your vital life force and your ability to heal yourself. You can use them safely and successfully to treat a wide range of common ailments. Individual remedies are made either from the whole plant or from just a part of it. This insures against unpleasant side effects that may occur when an active substance is isolated and prescribed in concentrated doses, as in modern medicine.

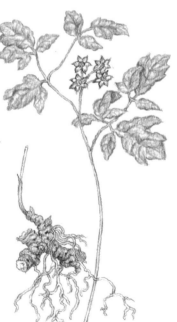

What to expect

When you first consult a herbalist, you will be asked for details of your medical history and then given a full physical examination, covering blood pressure, pulse, and heart rate. You may also be asked questions about your emotional state.

Blue cohosh

Some medicinal herbs have potent effects and need to be prescribed by a practitioner. A tonic of the herbs cramp bark, false unicorn root, blue cohosh, and squaw vine, for example, may be used effectively during the last three months of pregnancy to prepare the uterus and cervix for birth. However, several of the herbs have powerful effects on the body and so the tonic must be taken only on prescription.

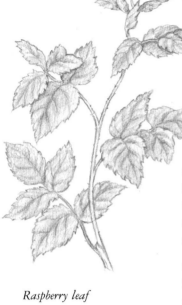

Many herbalists have their own pharmacies and will make up ointments, tonics, and tinctures, and supply dried herbs to match their own prescriptions. You can pick some of the commoner herbs and use them fresh or dried to make infusions or decoctions, two of the commonest ways in which herbal remedies are taken in the home. It is important, however, to keep to recommended dosages, since strong and mild infusions of the same herb may have quite different effects.

To make a mild infusion, use 14g (½ oz) of the dried leaves, flowers, or stems of a plant, or 28g (1oz) of fresh. Pour 560ml (1 pint) of boiling water over the herb, stir the mixture, and leave it to stand for 10 to 15 minutes before drinking. To make a decoction, use 28g (1oz) of the dried woody stems, roots, nuts or seeds, either ground to a powder or broken into little pieces. Use double the quantity if fresh. Add 840ml (1½ pt) of cold water, bring the mixture to the boil, and simmer for about 20 to 30 minutes until the water is reduced and any roots are soft. Herbs may also be taken in tablet, syrup, or tincture form, used externally in the bath, or applied as ointments, creams, compresses, or poultices.

Caution: All the herbs recommended in this book have been tried and tested for use in pregnancy but it is wise, nevertheless, to consult a herbalist if you are in any way uncertain about self-help treatment. It is important to tell your doctor of any herbal remedies that you intend to take.

Raspberry leaf

The following herbal teas are available in health-food stores and make delicious, health-giving substitutes for tea and coffee in pregnancy. It is wise, however, to vary your choice of herbal teas and to avoid drinking large quantities of any one infusion in a day:

Red raspberry leaf tea is extremely beneficial in the last three months of pregnancy and helps to tonify the uterus

Chamomile tea is calming, induces sleep, and aids digestion

Limeflower tea is soothing and sleep-inducing

Peppermint tea is stimulating, a tonic, and a digestive, but should not be drunk when you are taking homeopathic remedies

Lemon verbena tea is mildly stimulating and refreshing

Nettle tea is rich in iron and is a blood purifier, and an excellent tonic in pregnancy. It eases leg cramps and strengthens the kidneys

Fennel tea, slippery elm tea, and Japanese hancha or kukicha tea can calm the stomach and aid digestion

Mu tea increases vitality and strength

Dandelion root coffee acts as a mild diuretic and cleansing liver tonic

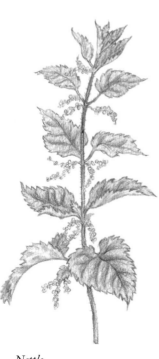

Nettle

Caution: When taken in excess, German chamomile can cause vomiting.

Bach flower remedies

Bach flower remedies are prescribed according to emotional state rather than physical symptoms, in the belief that the basis of disease lies in the mind or spirit and that healing will occur spontaneously once the mental state improves. The 38 remedies, each containing the essential properties of different wild flowers or plants, were formulated by Edward Bach, a Welsh doctor, in about 1930. They are grouped according to their effectiveness in coping with a predominant emotion; for example, loneliness, fear, uncertainty, despondency, grief, anger, guilt, or shock.

What to expect

You may be able to treat your complaint successfully with the help of a book describing the uses of the individual flower remedies, but if you are at all uncertain, consult a practitioner. All of the remedies are harmless and may be safely taken throughout pregnancy. They are prescribed in dilute form like homeopathic remedies, in a little alcohol. Either add four drops to a glass of water and sip slowly, or use the dropper provided to place a few drops on your tongue, behind your ears, and on the pulse points in your wrists. You may need to take the flower remedies regularly for several weeks for treatment to be effective.

Rescue Remedy is a marvellous emergency treatment, containing cherry plum, clematis, impatiens, rock rose, and star of Bethlehem. It has an immediate effect after a shock or accident and is also useful in stressful situations. During pregnancy it is a good idea to keep some in your handbag and to take it whenever you feel queasy or faint. It is helpful for insomnia and may be taken in labour. As a cream, it does wonders for bites, stings, and burns, and may help ease rashes and itching skin.

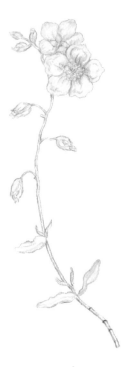

Rock rose

Homeopathy

Homeopathy was formulated by a German doctor, Samuel Hahnemann, in 1790. In contrast to orthodox medicine, homeopathy sees symptoms as positive attempts by the body to rid itself of disease. In consequence, it prescribes remedies to assist rather than to suppress symptoms. For example, where orthodox medicine might treat constipation with a laxative drug, homeopathy prescribes a minute dose of a substance that could cause constipation in a healthy person. In this way, the body is stimulated to react and release its own healing power. This approach is founded on the first principle of homeopathy, known as the law of similars, which states that any substance capable of making you ill may also cure you if administered in a small enough dose to treat the same symptoms.

The small dose, or minimum dose as it is otherwise known, is prepared by repeatedly diluting a substance and shaking it vigorously between each dilution. This shaking process, known as succussion, releases the healing power of the substance, while the dilution process eliminates side effects.

The more a remedy is diluted using this method of preparation, the more potent it becomes, so that only a minute quantity is needed to be effective. When a substance is diluted to 1 part in 99, it is called a 1C potency. The most commonly recommended potencies for home treatment are 6C (where the dilution process has taken place six times) and 6X; higher potencies such as 200, 1M or 10M need to be prescribed by a homeopath.

Homeopathic remedies are effective in treating nausea, vomiting, respiratory and digestive disorders, urinary problems, anaemia, fluid retention, high blood pressure, emotional difficulties, and a variety of other conditions. They may also be taken to help prepare your body for birth.

What to expect

On your first visit to a homeopath, you may be surprised by the number of questions you are asked. There are many possible remedies for each complaint and a homeopath must try to match different aspects of your condition, such as thirst, food preferences, mood, type of pain, and so on, before making a final choice. He or she may recommend a constitutional remedy that aims to raise your general level of health by taking your character and disposition into account in addition to your physical symptoms. In Chapter 6, the term **constitutional treatment** is used to refer to this form of prescribing.

To be effective, homeopathic remedies need to be taken correctly (see below) and for the right period of time. If your symptoms do not improve in response to a self-help treatment, it is advisable to consult a homeopath. Occasionally a remedy may cause symptoms to worsen temporarily. This is a good sign and you should stop taking a remedy at this point, since a steady improvement will generally follow. **Always seek the help of a professional homeopath if you are suffering from a chronic complaint, or if your symptoms are severe and do not respond readily to self-help treatment.**

Points to observe when using homeopathic remedies:

❖ Store remedies in a dark, cool place away from strong smells, such as camphor or eucalyptus

❖ Coffee and peppermint antidote some remedies and should be avoided during treatment

❖ Do not eat, drink (except water), or clean your teeth for 20 minutes before or after taking a remedy

❖ To take a pill, tip one from the bottle into the lid and then on to your own hand. You can handle the pill you are about to take but avoid handling one you are giving to someone else, and do not replace a pill in the container after it has been touched

❖ Place soft tablets or powders under the tongue and leave them to dissolve; suck hard tablets for a while and then chew them

❖ Do not take remedies of a higher potency than 30C without a prescription from a homeopath

Aromatherapy

Aromatherapy uses essential oils and massage to induce relaxation, raise the energy level, and restore balance to the mind, body, and soul. The oils are pure aromatic substances extracted from flowers, trees, fruits, and herbs. They are powerful, highly odorous, and volatile, and may be inhaled, used for massage, added to the bath water, applied as compresses, or used in vaporizers.

When inhaled, essential oils enter the body via the olfactory nerves in the nose, stimulating the part of your brain that regulates the nervous and hormonal systems. They also reach the bloodstream and internal organs via the lungs and skin. Some essential oils benefit the whole system, while others have quite specific uses. Neroli (orange blossom) and lavender help to promote new cell growth and for that reason are especially useful in pregnancy. Of the full range of essential oils available, many are used for their healing properties as antiseptics, detoxifiers, stimulants, digestives, or diuretics.

Aromatherapy is an excellent therapy for nervous exhaustion and stress due to the beneficial effects that essential oils have on the autonomic nervous system. It is also an effective treatment for conditions that can be influenced through the skin, respiratory problems, high blood pressure, insomnia, nausea, stretchmarks, fluid retention, cystitis, vaginal infections, and varicose veins. During pregnancy it is wise to consult a trained holistic aromatherapist, who will be qualified to treat a broad spectrum of health problems. Other aromatherapists may use essential oils for beauty therapy or general relaxation after a short training period of only three to four days but are not qualified to treat common ailments in pregnancy.

What to expect

A thorough case history will be taken at the start of a session and you will then be asked to undress and lie down, covered with a warm towel, on the massage couch. The therapist will choose a mixture of oils for you and may use different styles of massage, including shiatsu and reflexology, which are particularly effective in pregnancy. The depth of the massage and the parts of the body massaged will be chosen to suit your needs and comfort. Sometimes it will be suggested that you continue to use the oils at home. The prices of essential oils vary. Some are expensive but they are long lasting, since only small quantities are needed for each treatment. (see p. 93 for suppliers of oils).

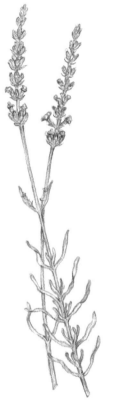

Lavender

A relaxing aromatic bath

Choose one or two of the following essential oils. Dilute a total of three or four drops in one tablespoon of milk or base oil, and add to your bath water:

lavender, sandalwood, geranium, rose, jasmine,
ylang-ylang, lemon, bergamot, orange, or rosewood

Caution: In pregnancy the following oils should be avoided: oreganum, clary sage, savory, thyme, wintergreen, basil, clove, hyssop, lemongrass, marjoram, myrrh, cinnamon bark, and pennyroyal.

Hypnotherapy

Hypnotherapy uses mental relaxation techniques to encourage the conscious mind to let go so that the unconscious becomes more open to suggestions from the therapist. It can help you to cope with pain and emotional problems, such as phobias, and may improve conditions that are worsened by stress. It may also be used effectively if you are trying to give up smoking or drinking alcohol, or to reduce fear of internal examinations.

What to expect

At the beginning of a session, a thorough case history will be taken, and you will then be asked to lie down. To relax you and induce a trance, the therapist will talk slowly, encouraging you to concentrate on a visual image, to imagine a downward movement, or to follow a counting sequence. He or she may then make positive suggestions to help you find a way to overcome your problem. You will then be gently roused from the trance feeling calm and relaxed. Self-hypnosis may be taught for home use.

Psychotherapy or counselling

Psychotherapy or counselling may be recommended to help you deal with emotional problems. These may stem from intrauterine life, birth, infancy, or childhood, from a crisis or conflict in your present situation, or from anxiety about the future.

Counsellors are usually specialized in particular areas – for example, marriage guidance or childbirth – and may offer advice to help you overcome a specific problem. Psychotherapy differs from counselling in that the therapist is trained to provide a context in which you can explore your emotional life in depth. This involves establishing a constant, secure relationship in which there is enough trust for you to release your innermost feelings so that healing can take place. In pregnancy, therapy can be invaluable in helping you to sort out confusion and to come to terms with yourself, and may effectively prevent a depression occurring later on.

There are, however, many different types of therapy and you may need to do quite a bit of research before finding the one that is right for you.

What to expect

A counselling session involves an informal discussion, in which you are free to express your feelings. In response, the counsellor may make helpful suggestions. Usually more than one session is needed.

During a psychotherapy session, you may sit or lie down. Most therapists adopt the technique of "mindful presence", remaining attentive and supportive so that healing can take place in its own space and time. Some therapists use bodywork or breathing techniques to assist the release of feelings. Sessions are regular and this therapy, which is often long term, can produce profoundly positive results when successful.

CHAPTER 6

HOLISTIC HEALING

While pregnancy is usually a time of great health and vitality, discomforts or problems can arise which may be successfully treated with self-help or by consulting a complementary therapy practitioner. Natural remedies can sometimes offer a safe, chemical-free alternative to orthodox medical treatment, and may be used to complement your antenatal care. Always discuss any self-help treatment you are considering with your midwife or doctor, and seek diagnosis and professional help by a trained expert if necessary. If you have one of the ailments listed below, turn to the relevant page.

You will find some self-help suggestions and advice about which therapies may be helpful for professional treatment. Several alternatives are given, so begin with the one that appeals to you most, and start by reading about how the therapy works in Chapter 5. If you have chosen the right treatment you should see signs of improvement after a week or so, unless your therapist tells you that several treatments will be needed before you can expect a positive response. It is not unusual to experiment with a few, before finding the treatment that works best for you. You may be able to combine therapies successfully, but it is usually best to do this with the guidance of an experienced therapist.

CONTENTS

For ease of reference, the index of ailments below is listed in alphabetical order. Within the chapter, the individual ailments are grouped loosely under related body systems.

Anxiety

Some degree of anxiety is a normal part of everyday life and to be expected as you approach the challenges of birth and parenthood. Persistent feelings of uncertainty, worry, or fear, however, need to be acknowledged, and taken seriously.

Anxiety may give rise to a range of symptoms including headaches, muscular tensions, digestive disorders, skin rashes, infections, high blood pressure, insomnia, depression, heart palpitations, panic attacks, or phobias. The cause of your anxiety may lie in past experiences, present sources of conflict, or uncertainty about the future.

Professional treatment *Counselling* or *psychotherapy* If your anxiety is severe, it is important to seek the help of a counsellor or psychotherapist. *Cranial osteopathy* When combined with psychotherapy, this treatment can help to release suppressed feelings. *Acupuncture* Regular sessions of this therapy will balance the energies and alleviate symptoms. *Hypnotherapy* Positive suggestions made under hypnosis may be helpful but should be combined with adequate counselling. *Homeopathy* To find the right remedy for your particular symptoms, it is essential to consult a homeopath. If you are run down or ner-vous, homeopathic tissue salts may be prescribed and, if taken on a regular basis, can be extremely effective. *Bach flower remedies* If prescribed and taken regularly, certain of the Bach flower remedies may help to relieve anxiety.

Self-help suggestions Try to get to the bottom of what is worrying you by talking things through with your partner or someone close to you. Allow your feelings to surface, and make a conscious effort to reduce any stress in your present situation. Exercise regularly (see pp. 30-41), and set aside time for deep breathing, meditation, and relaxation (see pp. 18-21 and 42). Eat a healthy, balanced diet (see pp. 22-29) and drink soothing herbal teas of chamomile (see *caution,* p. 63) or limeflower daily. *Homeopathy* If you are fearful, take one tablet of Aconite 30C to alleviate symptoms. Repeat half an hour later if necessary. *Aromatherapy* For a relaxing bath, add two or three drops of essential oil of chamomile, lavender, bergamot, melissa, rose, or geranium to the water, or a combination of two or three of these oils. *Shiatsu* Applying pressure to the points illustrated below may bring relief. Either shiatsu the point yourself, or ask your partner to do so.

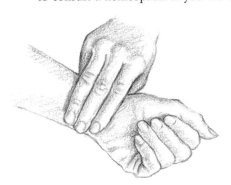

Shiatsu
a) Locate the point Pericardium 6 (PC6) by measuring three fingers' width from the first wrist crease on the inside of your arm. The point lies at this distance from the wrist between the two tendons.

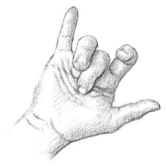

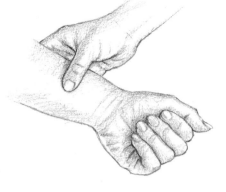

b) Using your thumb, press firmly on the point Pericardium 6 (PC6). Continue pressing for 5-7 seconds. Repeat 3 times. Locate the point on your other arm in the same way, measuring three fingers' width from the wrist crease. Press the point firmly for 5-7 seconds. Repeat 3 times.

c) Locate the point Pericardium 8 (PC8) by bending your middle finger until it touches the centre of your palm. Press firmly on the point and hold for 5-7 seconds. Repeat 3 times. Locate and shiatsu the same point on your other hand for 5-7 seconds. Repeat 3 times.

Depression

If you are deeply unhappy or depressed, your symptoms may include low energy, little inclination to get up in the morning or do anything, excessive weeping, a gloomy outlook on life, and lack of appetite. Emotionally, you may feel confused and despondent, sad, or even angry and frustrated. It is important to seek help, both for your own sake and for that of your unborn child.

Deep depression usually has its roots in past experiences or traumas that have not been properly understood or resolved, and about which feelings may have been suppressed. Alternatively, something in your present situation may be making you depressed; an illness or death in the family, for example, or difficulties in your relationship with the baby's father. Other possible causes include loneliness, financial problems, and food allergy (see p.71).

Professional treatment *Psychotherapy* A skilled therapist whom you like and trust can help you to release feelings, unravel confusion, and resolve conflicts.

Regular sessions on an ongoing basis may be necessary. **Try to avoid anti-depressant drugs or tranquillizers since these may harm your baby.** *Cranial osteopathy, Acupuncture, Homeopathy, Herbalism,* or *Aromatherapy* Any of these therapies can be helpful when combined with psychotherapy.

Self-help suggestions Talking to a close friend, relative, childbirth educator, or midwife can go a long way to helping you through a depression. Try to eat a healthy, balanced diet (see pp. 22-29) and take plenty of rest. Relaxation techniques, such as deep breathing and meditation (see pp. 18-21), combined with regular exercise (see pp. 30-43) can help to improve the way you feel. *Bach flower remedies* Individual remedies may alleviate the symptoms of depression. Always obtain professional advice when using the remedies. *Aromatherapy* Essential oils such as bergamot, jasmine, neroli, or rose are generally uplifting. Add two or three drops of one or a combination of two of the oils to your bath water.

Tiredness

During the early stages when your body is accommodating the physical changes of pregnancy, you may become easily exhausted. You should grow stronger in the months that follow but may need to rest more frequently again toward full term. During these last few months you may find it difficult to get comfortable at night and your sleep may be interrupted by the urge to urinate. Continuous tiredness, however, is unusual and may be caused by pain, anaemia, depression, anxiety, or insomnia.

Professional treatment Consult your doctor to establish the cause of your fatigue. Treat any aches or pains that may be causing the tiredness (see pp. 83-4). *Acupuncture, Shiatsu,* or *Aromatherapy* These therapies are effective in balancing and releasing the energy flow and reducing fatigue.

Self-help suggestions Sleep as much as you are able to and rest during the day. Eat well, avoiding junk foods, and don't worry about weight gain, unless it is excessive (see p. 82), since you will lose it naturally after the birth. If you find it difficult to eat three

meals a day, compensate by eating smaller, more frequent meals. An organic multivitamin and mineral tonic and a B vitamin complex are useful supplements, while royal jelly is a valuable energy booster and a good general tonic in pregnancy. Practise yoga daily (see pp. 30-43) and take plenty of fresh air, gently increasing your level of exercise by walking and swimming regularly. Massage on a regular basis (see pp. 44-55) will help to stimulate your energy flow. *Homeopathy* Take Kali phos 6X three times daily for up to a week. If there is no improvement, consult a skilled homeopath.

A relaxing massage oil

50ml (1¾ oz) of grapeseed or almond oil
essential oils of bergamot, geranium, and sandalwood

Add 12 drops of the essential oil of bergamot, 4 drops of geranium, and 9 drops of sandalwood to your choice of base oil. Use with a full body massage (see pp. 52-53) before going to sleep.

Insomnia

The odd sleepless night is common in pregnancy, but insomnia can be exhausting if it persists. Its causes may be deep seated and linked to anxiety or depression, or it may occur for more obvious reasons, such as indigestion, overstimulation, discomfort, pain, or the need to urinate, with a cycle of sleeplessness and worry causing its recurrence.

Professional treatment If an emotional problem seems to be at the root of your insomnia, follow the treatment and self-help guidelines given for anxiety and depression on the previous two pages. *Hypnotherapy* A skilled hypnotherapist can teach you to induce sleep by self-hypnosis, and may also help you to release suppressed emotions. *Acupuncture* An effective treatment for insomnia and a useful substitute for sleeping pills, acupuncture balances the energy and treats those parts of the body depleted by sleeplessness.

Self-help suggestions Eat several hours before bedtime, making sure your meal is easily digestible. Avoid stimulants such as tea and coffee; a soothing herbal infusion of chamomile (see *caution*, p. 63) or limeflower makes a good substitute. Before going to bed, try taking a calcium and magnesium supplement or a calcium-rich drink such as warm milk to help you sleep.

Make sure your room is well ventilated and your bed comfortable. Use extra pillows if necessary (see p. 42). Before sleep, do the sequence of exercises on pages 32-41, and follow this with a relaxing bath. Massage of the head and neck will help to relieve tension (see pp. 50-51).

Homeopathy Take a combination remedy of Avena sativa, Passiflora and Valeriana (see *Useful Addresses*, p. 93 for suppliers of homeopathic remedies) before going to bed and another if you wake up during the night. If insomnia is persistent, consult a professional homeopath. *Bach flower remedies* A few drops of Rescue Remedy in a little warm water may help to relax you if you are wakeful. *Aromatherapy* Add two or three drops of the sleep-inducing essential oil of lavender to a base oil and use it with a massage before bed. Or try a hot footbath containing lavender oil to encourage energy to drain from the head so that sleep comes easier. *Herbalism* Take 1 tablet of Valerian or Passiflora before bedtime to calm and relax you and encourage sound sleep.

Allergies

In pregnancy, an allergy can become apparent for the first time and may be the cause of a wide range of symptoms. Irritations of the skin and mucous membrane are common allergic reactions. However, if you suffer from severe digestive disturbances such as heartburn, diarrhoea, or constipation, recurrent cystitis, or colds that won't clear up, you may find that an allergy is the cause. Other problems such as depression, tiredness, insomnia, migraine, headaches, and asthma can also be allergic reactions.

If you develop an allergy, you may be intolerant of a specific substance (the allergen) in your environment or diet. Among the commonest allergens are house mites in dust and animal fur, pollen, food additives, dairy products, wheat, eggs, coffee, oranges, and certain laundry detergents and cosmetics.

Prevention Eat a healthy balanced diet, containing plenty of fresh, whole foods (see pp. 22-29), to help build up your resistance. Take one 15 to 30mg dose of the supplement zinc orotate at a different time of day from any iron supplements. Avoid using aluminium cooking pots since research has shown that these may be associated with allergies. If there is a history of allergy in your family, be sure to breastfeed after the birth for as long as possible since your milk contains immunoglobulins that will strengthen your baby's immunity to allergies.

Professional treatment If you think that you may be allergic, seek professional advice. Allergy tests or avoidance measures may be advised as a means of identifying the allergen. Alternatively, constitutional treatment may be adopted with the aim of improving your general health until symptoms recede. *Acupuncture, Homeopathy, Herbalism,* or *Aromatherapy.* These therapies may all be helpful in the treatment of allergies.

Self-help suggestions Once the cause of your allergy has been identified, you can take steps to eliminate it from your diet or immediate environment. If the allergen is a staple, such as wheat, eggs, or dairy products, you will need to adjust your diet with care. Take care to substitute foods that have the same nutritional value (see pp. 22-29), consulting a nutritionist if need be. Organic soya products and vegetable oils can take the place of dairy foods but make sure you have an adequate intake of calcium from other sources. Other grains can replace wheat, and vegetable protein makes a substitute for eggs. Additives are easily eliminated from the diet by eating fresh unprocessed food. If a laundry detergent or cosmetic is causing a reaction, you can buy biodegradable household products from health-food stores. Hypoallergenic cosmetics are stocked by most pharmacists. *Bach flower remedies* Rescue Cream can be applied locally to skin irritations.

Hay fever

If you suffer from hay fever, your symptoms may get worse while you are pregnant. Frequent sneezing, a runny or blocked nose, headaches, sore watery eyes, a sore throat, and a cough are all symptoms commonly associated with hay fever. These may affect you seasonally when the pollen count is high or throughout the year if you are allergic to something in your immediate environment (see *Allergies*, p. 71). Sometimes no obvious cause can be found.

Prevention *Homeopathy* If you are a seasonal sufferer, anticipate the months when the pollen count will be high and start taking a homeopathic hay fever remedy or tissue salts ahead of time. These are available from health-food stores and some pharmacists, or you can have them made up by a homeopathic pharmacy. To build up your resistance, take one 15 to 30mg dose of zinc orotate at a different time of day from any iron supplements.

Professional treatment *Homeopathy* if your hay fever is severe, consult a homeopath for constitutional treatment (see p. 65). Do so preferably before symptoms occur; for example, during the winter months if you are allergic to pollen.

Self-help suggestions Stay indoors when the pollen count is at its highest and avoid using antihistamines, since these will only suppress symptoms and are not recommended during pregnancy. Increasing the fibre content of your diet (see p. 24) and cutting down on dairy products may help to reduce mucus but make sure you eat other calcium-rich foods (see p. 25). Vitamin supplements C, A, E, and B complex are all helpful in allergic conditions. A solution of strong, cold chamomile tea (see *Eye problems*, p. 73) will soothe sore eyes. *Shiatsu* Ask your partner to apply pressure to the points illustrated below to relieve symptoms.

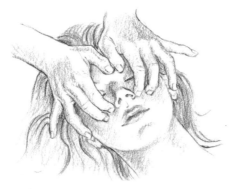

Shiatsu

a) Locate the points Large Intestine 20 (LI20) on either side of your nostrils at the top of the creases that run toward your mouth, and the points Stomach 3 (ST3) in the centre of your cheekbones. Using your index and middle fingers, shiatsu all four points at once, pressing down away from the nose. Hold for 5-7 seconds. Repeat 3 times.

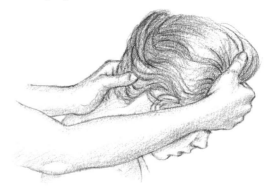

b) Helper: Locate the point Gall Bladder 20 (GB20) 2.5cm (1in) to the side of the midline of your partner's neck at the base of her skull. Rest your hand on the back of her neck and, using your thumb, shiatsu the point, pressing firmly upward into the bone. Hold for 5-7 seconds. Repeat 3 times. Change hands to shiatsu the same point on the other side of the midline.

Eye problems

Due to the hormones released in pregnancy, fluid in the eye tissues can increase, especially during the last three months, and may affect your sight. If you already wear glasses or contact lenses, your vision may be less focused for a while. All should return to normal after the birth so it is not worth changing your glasses. Be sure to inform your doctor immediately, however, if you see flashing lights or experience seriously blurred vision, since these symptoms may indicate more serious problems.

Self-help suggestions To revive tired eyes, make a soft fabric bag 15cm (6in) long and 5cm (2in) wide, and fill with 168g (6oz) of uncooked rice. Place gently over the eyes and relax. *Herbalism* Bathe infected eyes with a herbal eyewash made from golden seal roots and eyebright. Simmer 28g (1oz) of the dried roots in 560ml (1pt) of water for 10 to 15 minutes. Take off the heat and add one teaspoon of dried eyebright. Leave to cool and strain before using. Alternatively, add three or four drops of euphrasia tincture to an eggcupful of cooled, boiled water, and use the liquid to bathe the eyes. If there is no improvement after treatment with either of the above remedies, consult a herbal practitioner or your doctor. As a soothing remedy for tired eyes, soak cotton wool pads in cold chamomile tea and place them over your eyes. *Shiatsu* To relieve tired or swollen eyes, ask your partner to apply pressure to the points illustrated below or do so yourself.

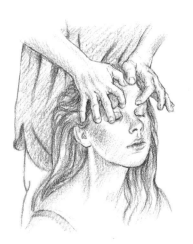

Shiatsu

a) Helper: Find the points Bladder 2 (BL2) on your partner's forehead at the start of each eyebrow. Using your index fingers, press up and out on the edge of each eye socket for 5-7 seconds. Repeat 3 times.

b) Helper: Support your partner's head against your thighs. Locate the point Gall Bladder 1 (GB1) in the depression at the corner of each eye. Using your index fingers press firmly for 5-7 seconds. Repeat 3 times.

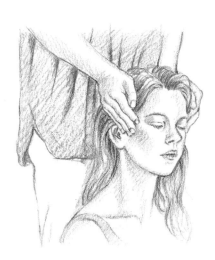

Teeth and gum problems

During pregnancy, your gums tend to swell and may bleed easily when brushed. If food particles become trapped between the teeth, this can give rise to infected gums – a condition known as gingivitis.

Prevention Eat a nutritious, wholefood diet (see pp. 22-29), including plenty of fresh, raw vegetables and fruit. Avoid sugary or highly refined foods and sweet, soft drinks. Brush your teeth after all meals with a soft brush, using a toothpaste that contains fluoride and making circular motions where the teeth meet the gums. Use dental floss or tooth picks to remove particles from between the teeth. See your dentist regularly but avoid X-rays.

Professional treatment *Bach flower remedies* If you need to see a dentist, take Rescue Remedy just before treatment. If a local anaesthetic is suggested, ask for the type that does not include adrenalin.

Self-help suggestions If your gums bleed when you brush your teeth, rinse your mouth with a solution of warm water and sea salt, then rub the gums with a little homeopathic hypercal tincture. Eat plenty of vitamin-C-rich foods and take vitamin C supplements. *Homeopathy* To soothe painful bruising after dental treatment, take Arnica 30C twice daily for one to two days. For shooting nerve pain, take Hypericum 30C twice daily for one to two days.

Sinusitis

A blocked nose is a common symptom in pregnancy. It results from an increase in fluid in the mucous membrane linings, which causes swelling and a blockage of the sinuses. If the blocked sinuses become infected, sinusitis may develop. This complaint is indicated by pain at the base of the nose and around the eyes, which worsens if the head is lowered, and stuffiness in the head. Headaches and fever may occur in acute cases.

Professional treatment *Osteopathy* This can be a remarkably effective treatment for painful sinusitis. *Acupuncture* This therapy may help to balance fluid circulation and reduce congestion in the sinuses.

Homeopathy Constitutional treatment (see p. 65) is recommended for chronic sinusitis.

Self-help suggestions Drink plenty of fluids and eat a lot of garlic and parsley, mixed in with your food. *Homeopathy* Take Silica 6X or Kali bichromicum 6X three times daily for up to a week, stopping when symptoms start to improve. Consult a homeopath if there is no improvement. *Aromatherapy* Make up the inhalation described under coughs and colds (see p. 75). Inhale to relieve symptoms, but do not use in combination with homeopathy. *Shiatsu* Apply pressure to the points illustrated under *Hay fever* (see p. 72) to bring relief.

Breathlessness

Breathlessness is common in pregnant women after mild physical exertion. If, however, you experience breathlessness at other times, this may mean that you are overweight, unfit, anaemic, or have a deficient diet, in which case you should consult your doctor and follow the advice given on pages 77 and 82. Breathlessness is more likely to occur in women who are expecting large babies or twins.

Self-help suggestions Eat a healthy, balanced diet (see pp. 22-29) and practise deep breathing and yoga daily (see pp. 18 and 30-43). Swimming is an excellent way to build up your stamina without strain. Gentle breaststroke while breathing calmly and deeply will reduce breathlessness. *Shiatsu* Applying pressure to the points illustrated below will help to tonify the chest.

Shiatsu

a) Helper: Support your partner's arm with one hand. Use your other hand to shiatsu with your thumb down the lung meridian (shown) that runs along the inside of the arm.

b) Helper: Support your partner's upper back with a large cushion and place another one under her knees. Locate the points Lung 1 (LU1) in the depressions below the collar bone on either side of her chest. Using your thumbs, press firmly on the points for 5-7 seconds. Repeat 3 times.

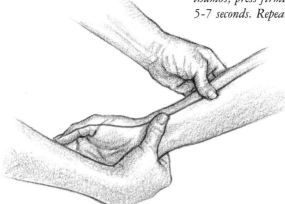

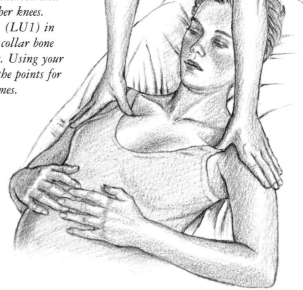

Coughs, colds, and chest infections

During pregnancy hormonal changes may cause swelling in the mucous membrane linings of the nasal passages and sinuses. As a result, coughs, colds, and bronchitis can be more difficult to clear than usual. They may be caused by infections, viruses, or, in some instances, allergies, but are more likely to occur if your vitality and resistance level are low. Colds that occur at the end of pregnancy tend to clear up during labour and are unlikely to prevent normal breathing during birth.

Prevention To build up your resistance, eat well, including vitamin C-rich foods (see p. 25), and make sure you get enough sleep. *Shiatsu* or *Acupuncture* Regular treatment with either of these therapies will improve your natural immunity to infection.

Self-help suggestions Eat garlic and onions or take garlic capsules to help combat the infection, and drink plenty of fluids. Zinc supplements and extra vitamin C will strengthen your resistance, and B vitamins are helpful if you are under stress. Use a humidifier if you have central heating. Try to remember to sit down and lean forward when coughing to reduce stress on your abdomen. *Homeopathy* At the first sign of a cold, take Aconite 30C every two hours for a period of 24 hours. If you develop a streaming headcold, take Allium cepa 30C three times daily until symptoms improve. Avoid using nasal drops or inhalants while taking homeopathic remedies. *Shiatsu* Applying pressure to the points recommended under *Hay fever* (see p. 72) will help to improve the flow of energy.

Aromatherapy inhalation for respiratory problems

essential oils of eucalyptus, lavender, lemon, and tea tree

Put 2 drops of each essential oil into a bowl of almost boiling water. Inhale the steam for 10 minutes.

Caution: do not use in conjunction with homeopathic remedies.

Herbal decoction for colds

4 cloves
1 tsp coriander seeds
2 cinnamon sticks (broken)
a few slices of ginger
840ml (1½ pt) of water
a slice of lemon
honey

Add the spices to the water. Bring to the boil and simmer for 20 minutes. Add the lemon and simmer for a further 5 minutes. Strain and sweeten with honey. Drink a hot cup of the mixture every 2 hours.

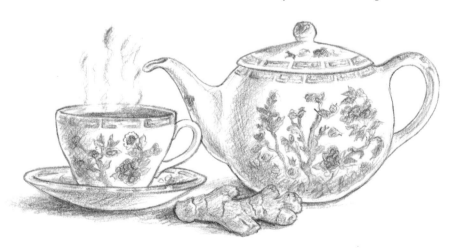

Skin changes

The blood supply to your skin increases while you are pregnant, resulting in a full, radiant, and healthy appearance. You will feel warmer and probably sweat more, and red spots or patches on the skin and flushed cheeks may also occur. Pigmentation can cause temporary darkening of nipples, areolae, birth marks, moles, and freckles, and a brown line called the "linea nigra" may appear down the centre of your belly. Sometimes, too, the colour of your face may darken. All of these changes are temporary and need no treatment. However, if moles increase in number during your pregnancy, you may find that some will remain after the birth.

If you suffer from acne, your symptoms may either get worse or improve while you are pregnant. Rashes and itching are common, especially during the last three months, and can cause discomfort and loss of sleep at night.

Self-help suggestions If you suffer from rashes or itching, you may find that your symptoms improve if you stop using soap. You can also try changing to a biodegradable laundry detergent. Wear cotton clothes to keep your skin cool. To soothe itching, fill a muslin cloth with a cupful of oatmeal, tie it up, and use it to wash yourself in the bath. Herbal chamomile (see *caution*, p. 63) and limeflower teas are soothing if taken last thing at night. *Herbalism* Use chickweed ointment to relieve an itchy rash. *Bach flower remedies* Rescue Cream may be helpful.

Inverted or flat nipples

An inverted nipple is dimple shaped and retracts rather than protrudes when the surrounding areola is compressed. Flat nipples are those that do not protrude or become erect when stimulated or cold. A truly inverted nipple is fairly rare and it is possible to have only one flat or inverted nipple. There are also different degrees of inversion ranging from slight, moderate to deep inversion. A midwife or breastfeeding counsellor (see *Useful Addresses,* p. 93, advice for breastfeeding mothers) will be able to help you to assess whether you have inverted nipples.

To test yourself, gently compress the areola with your fingers about 2.5cm (1in) behind the base of the nipple. If it protrudes it is not truly inverted. If it retracts or caves in then it may be inverted.

The main function of the nipple is to serve as a marker to help the baby to find the breast. It is important to be aware that babies do not feed from the nipple alone. Milk is made by the milk-producing cells in the breast tissue, and then pools in the little sinuses you can feel around the areola when the breasts are full. When feeding, the baby draws the nipple plus some of the surrounding breast tissue into the mouth. Shaped by the tongue, this forms a teat which reaches all the way to the back of the baby's throat when the baby is "latched on" properly. Then the baby's jaw and tongue movements guide the milk down the throat. The milk ejects spontaneously as a result of this stimulation, travelling from the milk sinuses through the teat formed by the baby and ejects through the openings in the nipple.

With a good "latch", the baby's mouth and gums will bypass the nipple and latch on to the areola. With persistence, patience, and good advice in the early days, most women can breastfeed successfully whatever the shape and size of the nipples, and the baby will help to draw out flat or inverted nipples.

Self-help suggestions Breastfeeding is a learned skill and it may take you and your baby time to get it right. Good positioning from the start will ensure that the baby "latches on" properly, so it is wise to arrange during late pregnancy for a breastfeeding counsellor to help you from the first day. It is now thought that massage techniques or wearing special breast shields to draw out the nipples in pregnancy are ineffectual. Spending some time with breastfeeding mothers while you are pregnant and observing how it is done is the best way to prepare.

Stretchmarks

In the early stages of pregnancy, reddish streaks, known as stretchmarks, may appear on the surface of the breasts as they gain in weight; in the later months weight gain on the buttocks and abdomen may give rise to stretchmarks in those areas. After birth, the marks will fade and become silvery white.

Prevention Stretchmarks may in some cases be prevented by using a good aromatic oil (see recipe right) daily from early on in pregnancy. You can also try taking a daily supplement of vitamin E to help increase elasticity. *Homeopathy* Take Calc fluor 6X three times daily for a week starting in early pregnancy; continue taking on alternate weeks for the rest of your pregnancy. This remedy will help to increase the tissue elasticity of dry or delicate skins.

Apply pure vitamin E oil locally to prevent or reduce scarring. Continue using regularly until after the birth.

Stretchmark prevention oil

50 ml (1¾ fl oz) of wheatgerm oil, or a mixture of wheatgerm and almond oil
essential oils of lavender and neroli

Fill a dark glass bottle with 50ml (1¾ fl oz) wheatgerm oil, or a mixture of wheatgerm and almond oil for a thinner solution. Add 3 drops of the essential oil of lavender and 15 drops of the essential oil of neroli. Massage daily after bathing.

Anaemia

If you are pale, tired, lethargic, lacking in appetite, and experience breathlessness on normal exertion, you may be suffering from anaemia.

During pregnancy your blood supplies not only your own body with oxygen but your baby's placenta as well. Oxygen is carried by a substance called haemoglobin found in the red blood cells. A slight drop in the concentration of haemoglobin in the blood is normal in pregnancy because of the general increase in fluid. If, however, your haemoglobin level falls below 10g per 100ml of blood, your body's ability to transfer oxygen may be reduced. If true anaemia occurs, treatment may be necessary.

Heavy menstrual bleeding prior to pregnancy or a diet deficient in the minerals and vitamins needed to make haemoglobin may both give rise to anaemia. Thalassaemia and sickle cell anaemia are inherited forms of the disease, common in women of African, West Indian, Mediterranean, or Asian origin. These types of anaemia need to be tested for in the early stages of pregnancy.

Prevention Prevention of anaemia is an important part of prenatal care and routine blood tests should be taken at around 16 and 30 weeks to assess your haemoglobin level. Make sure your diet contains all the minerals and vitamins needed to make haemoglobin – iron, zinc, cobalt, vitamin B1, vitamin B2, and folic acid – as well as vitamin C, which helps your body to absorb iron (see p. 25). After meals, drink herbal teas, such as nettle or raspberry leaf, which are rich in iron; avoid tea and coffee, which both reduce iron absorption. Supplement your diet with an organic multivitamin and mineral tonic, available from health-food stores.

Professional treatment *Herbalism* A tonic of yellow dock root, made up by a herbalist, is an effective way of raising the haemoglobin level, since the roots contain iron and the minerals and vitamins needed to absorb it. Follow the dosage prescribed.

Self-help suggestions Synthetic supplements of iron are often prescribed by doctors for anaemia, but they tend to cause constipation or heartburn and, unless zinc is taken at a different time of day from the iron, can create a zinc deficiency. They are also poorly absorbed by the system and may stress the bowels. As a safe, effective alternative, take double the recommended dose of an organic multivitamin and mineral tonic and a daily multivitamin tablet.

Supplement your diet with foods rich in iron (see p. 25). Eating them in combination with vitamin-C-rich foods on an empty stomach will assist iron absorption. Try to use cast-iron cookware since this will increase the iron content of your food. *Homeopathy* Take Ferrum metallicum 30C morning and night for two days to increase the iron in your blood. Then take Ferrum phosphoricum and Calcarea phosphoricum combined remedy 6X three times a day for two weeks (see *Useful Addresses*, p. 93 for suppliers of homeopathic remedies). This will improve your body's ability to absorb iron. After two weeks of this treatment, ask for a further blood test. If your haemoglobin level has failed to rise, your doctor may recommend another form of treatment.

Herbal tonic to prevent anaemia

15g (½ oz) each of the following dried herbs:
nettle leaves
parsley leaves
yellow dock root
peppermint leaves
2.25l (4pt) water

Place the dried ingredients in a heatproof jar (omitting the peppermint if you are also taking a homeopathic remedy). Fill with boiling water and steep for at least 8 hours. Strain and drink up to 4 cups a day until finished. Make a fresh infusion at the beginning of each month.

Caution: this tonic is used to prevent anaemia. If you are already anaemic, consult a herbalist.

Low blood pressure and fainting

While low blood pressure is often associated with good health, a sudden drop may cause fainting or dizziness. Fainting is fairly common in early pregnancy when softening of the muscular walls of the veins can cause blood to pool in the legs and the brain to become temporarily short of oxygen. You may feel faint after lying on your back or standing for too long, or after a hot bath; a sudden change of position or extreme heat can also cause faintness. Apart from the risk of injury, fainting is not usually a cause for concern, unless the fall in your blood pressure is extreme. However, you should inform your doctor.

Prevention While standing, you can practise contracting and relaxing your leg and buttock muscles to help the blood return to your head. When resting, lie on your side rather than your back. If you feel faint, sit down quickly to save yourself from injury. Put your head lower than your body or kneel on all fours until you feel better. *Bach flower remedies* Take a few drops of undiluted Rescue Remedy whenever you start to feel faint. *Homeopathy* Constitutional treatment (see p. 65) is beneficial in severe cases. *Shiatsu* Apply pressure to the fainting revival points illustrated, or ask your partner to do so.

Shiatsu
Helper: Locate the point Lung 9 (LU9) in the depression on the thumb side of the wrist crease. Next find the point Heart 7 (HT7) in the depression on the inside of the tendon on the little finger side. Shiatsu both points for 5-7 seconds. Repeat 3 times. Shiatsu the same points on the other arm. To treat yourself, press the points separately.

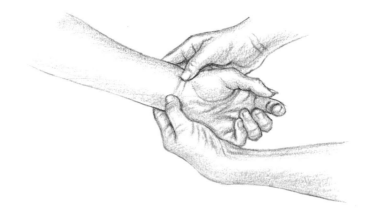

High blood pressure

High blood pressure may be physiological in some women in late pregnancy, or it may be a reaction to stress or anxiety. In very rare cases, it may result from hereditary or kidney disease.

Your blood pressure will be taken regularly to check that the systolic/diastolic pressure is within the normal range for pregnancy of between 110/70 and 140/90. The systolic figure is a measure of the pressure generated by your heart as it pumps blood around your body. The diastolic figure denotes the pressure in your arteries when your heart is at rest. A mild rise to below 150/100 may occur and while this usually poses no risk to mother or baby, frequent checking is necessary to ensure that pre-eclampsia (see below) does not develop. If your blood pressure rises more than 20 points, this may be a cause for concern and you should take advice from your doctor.

If high blood pressure is accompanied by swelling (see *Oedema,* p. 82) and protein in the urine, you may have pre-eclampsia. While you may feel perfectly well, this condition is potentially dangerous since it can develop into eclampsia, which is life-threatening. The causes of pre-eclampsia are unknown, although poor nutrition in pregnancy is thought to be a contributory factor.

Prevention Exercise regularly (see pp. 30-43) and eat a healthy, balanced diet, containing plenty of fresh raw fruit and vegetables (see pp. 22-29). Limiting your intake of red meat may help to reduce high blood pressure, but make sure you obtain adequate protein from other sources (see p. 26). Avoid emotional stress and stimulants, such as tea and coffee. Drink nettle, raspberry leaf, limeflower, and dandelion leaf teas.

Professional treatment There are effective natural alternatives to anti-hypertensive drugs, but be sure to inform your doctor of any treatment you are considering. Professional guidance and regular monitoring of your blood pressure and the protein in your urine are essential if you suffer from high blood pressure. *Herbalism* Many herbal tinctures help to reduce blood pressure, in particular those made with hawthorn flowers, leaves, or berries, but you will need to consult a herbalist. *Homeopathy* and *Acupuncture* Both these therapies are excellent for treating high blood pressure and pre-eclampsia, and can be successfully combined.

Self-help suggestions Plenty of rest and regular practice of the yoga exercises in Chapter 3 will help you keep your blood pressure down. Make sure you are eating enough protein and also foods high in calcium (see p. 25). Use salt moderately to taste but do not cut it out of your diet altogether. Eat plenty of garlic and onion or take garlic capsules daily, and add fresh celery to your diet. Cucumbers also help to reduce high blood pressure – either eat a whole cucumber or take half a cup of its juice daily. *Herbalism* Drink a calming infusion of passionflower, or passiflora, three times daily, using one teaspoon of the dried herb to a cup of water. Stop taking the infusion as soon as symptoms improve; if there is no improvement after a week, consult a herbalist.

If you develop pre-eclampsia, include potassium-rich foods such as bananas and lightly cooked potato peel in your diet, but avoid using potatoes with sprouts or green or dark brown patches. Drink raw beetroot/beets' juice daily or make up a salad of apple and grated beetroot/beets. Vitamin B complex taken on a daily basis together with 100mg of B6 or brewer's yeast may help to reduce high blood pressure. Alternatively, you can boost your diet with spirulina powder, a highly nutritious seaweed available from health-food stores. Adding young dandelion leaves, which are an excellent source of calcium and potassium, to your salads will vitalize your kidneys and help to reduce oedema.

Varicosities

During pregnancy, the increase in blood volume puts pressure on the veins, and hormonal secretions relax the walls of the blood vessels, making it more difficult for blood to return from the lower body back up to the heart. The weight of the enlarging uterus can put additional stress on the pelvic veins and constipation may also obstruct pelvic circulation. As a result, blood may pool in the lower body and varicose veins may appear on the legs, or in the vulva, or rectum. They can be unsightly, painful, and itchy. Those that appear in the rectum are commonly known as haemorrhoids or piles.

A tendency to varicosities may be hereditary but in pregnancy they are more common in women who have to stand for long periods or in those who are expecting twins. Vulval varicosities will usually disappear after the birth; varicose veins in the legs may or may not improve, although they are more likely to do so if given early treatment.

Prevention Eat well, including plenty of fibre in your diet (see pp. 22-29), and exercise regularly (see pp. 30-43) to encourage the smooth functioning of both your circulatory and eliminatory systems. Do the pelvic floor and inner thigh stretch exercises on pages 40 and 41.

Professional treatment *Herbalism* Herbs such as horse chestnut, nettle, yarrow, St. John's wort, and shepherd's purse help to improve blood flow, but must be prescribed by a herbalist. An ointment of either comfrey, yellow dock root, plantain, or yarrow, made up by a herbalist, may help to stop bleeding, reduce swelling, and ease pain. *Acupuncture* or *Shiatsu* Both these therapies may improve blood circulation. *Aromatherapy* This therapy can be effective in the treatment of varicose veins, but consultation with an aromatherapist is recommended in pregnancy. Essential oils may be prescribed for massage or for external application in compress form.

Self-help suggestions Varicosities can be helped in many ways and as individual women respond differently to the variety of treatments available, I have included a wide range of suggestions to choose from.

Avoid squatting or standing for long periods and, when you sit, never cross your legs. Instead, put them up whenever you can. Raise the foot of your bed 7.5 to 10cm (3 to 4in) and, if you wear support stockings, put your legs up for a while before putting them on. Walk, swim, and regularly work through the exercises on pages 30-43, paying heed to any cautionary advice. The best exercise for varicose veins is the inner thigh stretch exercise on page 41. Practise this twice daily, and while in the position, pump your calf muscles by alternating pointing your toes with extending your heels. This will assist the venous return. The pelvic floor exercise on page 40 is also helpful and should be done twice daily. If you suffer from haemorrhoids, tightening and releasing the muscles around the anal sphincter up to 50 times in quick succession will help to firm up the muscle

tone of the anal vessels. It is easy to get into the habit of doing this in bed first thing in the morning and last thing at night, adopting the knee-chest position (see p. 40, pelvic floor exercise, position *b*).

Eat raw garlic, onions, and parsley to increase the elasticity of your veins, and avoid constipation (see p. 87 for dietary advice). Sunflower seeds and wheatgerm are rich in vitamin E, a deficiency of which is linked with varicosities. A daily vitamin E supplement of up to 600 IU is recommended to help repair broken capillaries. Rutin supplements will build up the walls of the veins but should not be taken until the fourth month of pregnancy. Buckwheat is a good source of rutin that you can include in your diet.

Increasing your intake of vitamin-C-rich foods will promote healing and strengthen blood vessels, and raw beetroot/beets, either grated or as a juice, will fortify the liver and aid elimination. It is best to avoid spicy foods and aloe vera products.

To ease pain and reduce swelling, apply witch hazel on a lint compress to affected areas. Lemon juice or cider vinegar can be used instead but both may sting a little. Applications of grated raw potato are particularly effective for haemorrhoids and vulval varicosities, and you may also find it helpful to apply ice compresses to the perineum and anus. Taking a cold shower and directing the water up between the legs may help to relieve varicose veins. *Homeopathy* For haemorrhoids or painful varicose veins, take Hamamelis 6X three times daily for up to a week, stopping if symptoms improve. If there is no improvement, consult a homeopath. Calcarea fluorica 6X is good for building up elastic tissues and preventing recurrence. Take three times daily for up to a week. For external application, use one tablespoon of arnica tincture or lotion diluted in a litre (1¾ pt) of cold water. Apply twice daily to affected areas, using a saturated washcloth. *Herbalism* Horse chestnut ointment may be applied locally.

Herbal sitting bath for haemorrhoids

120g (4oz) of dried witch hazel
60g (2oz) of comfrey root
2.25l (4pt) of water

Steep the witch hazel and comfrey root in the water and simmer for 8 hours. Strain into a shallow bowl and discard the herbs. Sit in the solution for 15 minutes at least twice a day. Dry the genital area thoroughly after use. The solution can be re-used and is soothing even when haemorrhoids are severe.

Palpitations

During pregnancy, the volume of blood being pumped around the body increases and the heart has to work harder. Rapid or irregular beating of the heart is common at this time and usually not a cause for worry. Occasionally, however, anaemia (see p. 77) or anxiety (see p. 69) may be the cause, in which case it is best to talk to your doctor.

Self-help suggestions Exercise regularly (see pp. 30-41) and practise deep breathing, meditation, and relaxation (see pp. 18-21 and 42). *Bach flower remedies* When palpitations occur, take a dropperful of Rescue Remedy. *Shiatsu* Applying pressure to point PC6 (see *Anxiety*, p. 69) may bring relief. If you are anxious, follow the advice given on page 69.

Carpal tunnel syndrome

During pregnancy an increased supply of fluid to the extremities can cause swelling and pressure on the nerves and blood vessels which pass through the wrist canal, known as the carpal tunnel. As a result you may experience numbness, tingling, or pain in the hand and fingers and sometimes the arm. After pregnancy, the condition usually improves.

Professional treatment *Osteopathy* or *Acupuncture* Both these therapies may help to relieve numbness or pain. *Homeopathy* If your symptoms are severe, a skilled

homeopath may be able to recommend effective treatment for fluid retention.

Self-help suggestions Massage and exercise the hands, fingers, and wrists as illustrated below to help reduce fluid. Regular release of tension in the neck and shoulders through yoga or massage (see pp. 37 and 49-51) may also help. *Homeopathy* Take Ruta 30C three times daily for one week. *Shiatsu* Apply pressure to point PC6 (see *Anxiety*, p. 69) or, if you have pain in the thumb, press the point illustrated below.

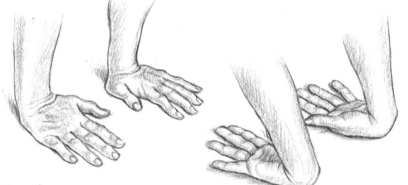

Massage
Helper: with your thumbs, massage your partner's wrists in the direction of the arrows. To massage yourself, stroke down one arrow at a time.

Shiatsu
Locate the point Lung 10 (LU10) in the centre of the mound at the base of your thumb. Press firmly and hold for 5-7 seconds. Repeat 3 times.

Exercise
a) Kneel on your hands and knees with your palms flat and fingers spread out. Lean your weight forward to gently stretch the inside of your wrists. Hold for a few seconds.

b) Lift your hands and bend the wrists so that you are able to place the backs of your hands on the floor. Gently lean back to stretch the outside of the wrists. Hold for a few seconds.

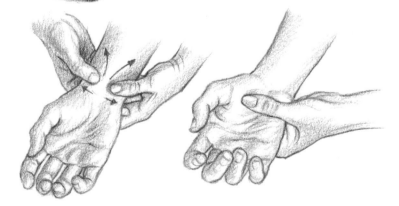

Oedema

In some women, a certain amount of puffiness, or swelling is normal in pregnancy and is caused by a general increase in fluid volume. Puffiness usually occurs in the feet, calves, ankles, fingers, and sometimes in the face. Hot weather, prolonged standing, and fatigue may make it worse, but you need only be concerned if white indentations marks, known as "pitting" occur when you apply finger pressure. If true "pitting" oedema is linked with high blood pressure and protein in the urine, this may be a sign of pre-eclampsia (see p. 79).

Prevention Eat a healthy, balanced diet (see pp. 22-29), take plenty of exercise (see pp. 30-41), and drink plenty of fluids. Avoid overeating and over-exerting yourself, and set aside time during the day to rest and relax (see p. 42).

Professional treatment *Herbalism* Dandelion leaves, golden rod, corn silk, and couch grass are gentle diuretics that need to be prescribed by a herbalist. *Homeopathy* Constitutional treatment (see p. 65) is recommended for oedema. *Acupuncture* This therapy can bring relief. *Aromatherapy* Massage with essential oils may also be helpful.

Self-help suggestions Rest with your feet up at intervals throughout the day, and sit rather than stand whenever you can. You may also find it helpful to practise the inner thigh stretch exercise on page 41. Supplement your diet with brewer's yeast, garlic, raw onions, apples, and red grapes or grape juice. *Homeopathy* Try taking Natrum muriaticum 6X three times daily for up to a week until symptoms improve. If they fail to do so, consult a homeopath.

Weight

Normal weight gain in pregnancy can be anything from 5kg (11lb) to 15kg (34lb). If your weight prior to pregnancy was normal, you should have little cause for worry provided you are eating well (see pp. 22-29), exercising regularly (see pp. 30-41), and are neither unduly tired nor breathless.

The weight that you put on is normally accounted for by the extra fat stores and fluid needed to cope with the demands of pregnancy, and the baby and placenta. However, excessive weight gain can occur and may prove difficult to lose.

If you put on less than 5kg (11lb), this may mean that you are losing weight or that your baby is not growing properly. One low reading should not necessarily be cause for concern, but your pregnancy may need to be carefully monitored if your baby appears to be "small for dates" on consecutive occasions. Small babies are usually strong and healthy, but it is wise to follow the self-help guidelines given below. If you were underweight prior to pregnancy, remember to inform your doctor. The growing foetus will very likely draw all it needs from your body, unless your own reserves are depleted.

Self-help suggestions for excessive weight gain Do not diet! Instead, concentrate your efforts on eating a healthy, balanced diet (see pp. 22-29). Make sure you are getting enough protein and wholegrain carbohy-drates but avoid sweet or fried foods, refined starches, and high calorie drinks. Eat plenty of fresh raw vegetables and fruit and some, but not too many, dried fruits since they can be fattening in excess. A good mineral and vitamin supplement may reduce cravings for refined, high-calorie foods. Non-strenuous exercise on a daily basis will help to burn up calories. Start gently with one or two exercises from the programme on pages 30-43 and gradually increase until you can do them all. Walk daily in the open air and try to go swimming one to three times a week.

Self-help suggestions for inadequate weight gain Improve your overall diet following the outlines given on pages 22-29 and do not diet on any account. If nausea is causing you to lose weight, try to eat small amounts of foods you can tolerate at regular intervals. Consult a nutritionist if you are seriously underweight. A vitamin B complex and Royal Jelly may increase your appetite, while an organic multivitamin and mineral tonic will boost your general health. If your baby is "small for dates", include zinc-rich foods (see p. 25) in your diet or take a daily supplement of zinc at a different time of day from any iron supplements. Make sure that you have adequate rest. *Counselling* If an emotional problem is the cause of your weight loss, seek the help of a skilled counsellor or therapist.

Pain

During pregnancy, your posture alters to accommodate the weight of your growing baby. In addition, the ligaments that hold the joints together are softened by hormonal secretions so that your skeleton increases in flexibility in preparation for birth. Most of the aches and pains experienced in pregnancy result from these changes and are usually not of a serious nature. However, underlying imbalances or unusual pressure on the nerves can result in discomfort or pain that may indicate a need for treatment. It is important to inform your doctor if you experience pain, especially if it is severe or persistent.

General advice on treating pain is given under the sections *Self-help suggestions* and *Professional treatment*. Individual aches and pains are listed under separate headings, together with exercises and other suggestions for treatment that may be helpful.

Prevention Practising the exercises on pages 30-41 will help both to alleviate and prevent many of the more common aches and pains.

Professional treatment *Osteopathy* or *Cranial osteopathy* Both these therapies can be successfully used to treat skeletal pain, and response to treatment in pregnancy is usually good. Make sure, however, that you consult an osteopath who is used to treating pregnant women. Your body is changing all the time, so you may need to return for regular sessions. *Acupuncture*

or *Shiatsu* These therapies may also bring relief. *Homeopathy* Consult a homeopath about remedies that you can use in conjunction with other therapies.

Self-help suggestions Avoid getting overtired or stressed. Pay attention to posture (see p. 34) and be sure not to aggravate your discomfort or pain by using your body unwisely. When lifting an object off the floor, squat down rather than bending forward and placing strain on your back. Sit rather than stand whenever possible. Regular swimming, especially toward the end of your pregnancy, and massage in the home may both help to relieve pain.

HEADACHES
In pregnancy, headaches may result from hormonal changes, tension, organ depletion, toxins, bad posture, or viral infections.

Self-help suggestions Soak a washcloth in cold water containing a few drops of essential oil of lavender. Apply this to the forehead and rest in a darkened room. Practising the sequence of exercises illustrated below will help both to relieve and prevent tension. *Aromatherapy* Massaging the spine, shoulders, neck, and head, using a massage oil containing a few drops of essential oil of lavender, may bring relief. Alternatively, place a few drops of essential oil of lavender in your bath water.

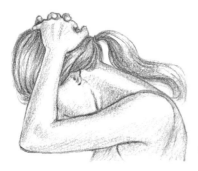
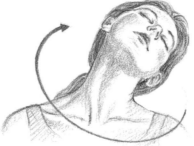
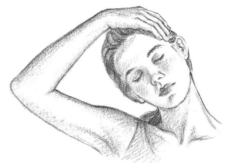

Exercise
a) Clasp your hands behind your head. Drop your chin and relax your arms. Breathe deeply, then slowly raise your head and let it hang back. Stretch the front of your neck by bringing your teeth together. Hold for a few seconds and come up slowly.

b) Relax your jaw and keeping your neck loose, slowly roll your head round in a complete circle, taking care to keep the rest of your body still. Breathe evenly and let your head roll round of its own momentum. Make 3 or 4 circles and then repeat in the other direction.

c) Let your head fall sideways toward your right shoulder. Place your right hand on top of your head and relax the arm. Breathe deeply. Hold for a few seconds. Repeat on the other side. Next, look over your right, then your left shoulder. Then shake your head slowly from side to side.

BACK PAIN

Pain in the lower back is common in pregnancy, since this is the area of the body most stressed by the additional weight you are carrying. However, you may also experience pain in the middle of the upper back, and in the neck and shoulders; this type of pain is generally caused by tension, or postural problems prior to pregnancy.

Self-help suggestions Practising the pelvic tuck in the exercise illustrated on page 39 will help relieve back pain and strengthen the spine. Remember to pay attention to your posture at all times (see p. 34), taking care not to arch your back and making sure you walk and stand with your feet parallel.

SACROILIAC PAIN

The hormonal secretions that soften the ligaments during pregnancy may also cause increased move-ment in the sacroiliac joints, which lie between the sacrum and iliac bones at the back of the pelvis. Pressure on the nerves, which stem from the lower part of the spine, can cause a shooting pain that may extend down the leg. The pain will be at its worst when you lie on your back, so try an alternative rest-ing position (see p. 42).

Professional treatment *Osteopathy* Treatment by an osteopath is essential, since sacroiliac pain drains the energy and may suddenly worsen.

Self-help suggestions concentrate on the exercises recommended for back pain (see above), but stop immediately if one of them causes you pain. The exercise illustrated below may help to relieve pain during a spasm.

RIB PAIN

Pain may be experienced on the side of the rib cage between the armpit and the waist. It usually occurs when the muscles of the diaphragm, which are attached to the ribs, and those of the abdomen are stretched and put under pressure by the expanding uterus. In later pregnancy your baby's movements may cause pain or considerable discomfort in the lower area of your rib cage.

Self-help suggestions Practising the shoulder stretch and inner thigh stretch exercises (see pp. 39 and 41) may bring relief.

PELVIC PAIN

In later pregnancy when the pubic joint expands in preparation for birth, pain in the front pubic area is common. It may worsen after walking or standing a lot, or when you are tired, so rest is essential.

Professional treatment *Osteopathy* Consult an osteopath to see whether you have a common condition called symphysis pubis dysfunction (see p. 85), and to relieve the symptoms.

ABDOMINAL PAIN

A variety of abdominal pains may be felt during pregnancy. They are usually associated with muscular changes or the growth of the uterus, and are rarely serious, often resembling a stitch or period pain in the lower abdomen. It is important, however, to inform your doctor. Severe or continuous pains require urgent medical attention.

Self-help suggestions Position yourself on all fours (see p. 38, position *c*). Relax and breathe deeply, releasing the abdominal muscles completely. Massage your belly gently if you feel this will help. Try using the same relaxation technique in the legs apart on the wall position (see p. 41, position *c*).

Exercise

Lie on your back with your knees bent, your feet a hips' width apart and parallel. Raise one knee and draw it gently toward your chest with your hands, keeping your hips parallel and your sacrum on the floor. Hold for a few seconds and repeat on the other side. If this exer-cise does not bring relief, consult an osteopath.

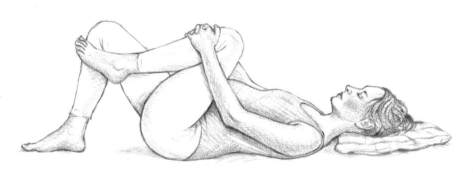

Symphysis pubis dysfunction (SPD)

In pregnancy, hormonal softening increases laxity of the tissues and there is a widening of the pubic joint in the front of the pelvis (symphysis pubis), designed to increase the pelvic diameters for birth. With SPD, increased laxity causes mild to severe pain which is felt in the front pubic area and is worse when walking, spreading the legs, lifting one leg, or moving in bed. There may also be associated pain in the lower back, sacroiliac joints, groin, or inner thighs. Postnatally, joint laxity will decrease again and, with the right care, further discomfort can be avoided.

Professional treatment *Physiotherapy* If SPD is causing you constant discomfort it is is essential to see a specialist at your local hospital to arrange to get a support belt for daytime use and a tubigrip bandage to use at night. If the pain is severe, it may be necessary to use elbow crutches for support when walking. *Osteopathy, Acupuncture,* or *Acupressure* and *Massage* These therapies can all bring great relief. It may be useful to rotate them if your symptoms are severe.

Self-help suggestions *Homeopathy* Take Sepia 30C three times daily for two days, then Arnica 30C and Hypericum 30C three times daily for five days. Repeat periodically. Reduce all weight bearing activities such as standing, walking, shopping, and lifting that are not essential, and rest a lot. Take great care when standing and walking to avoid turning out the feet, keeping them parallel instead, or even slightly

'pigeon toed'. (See exercise on p. 33.) Sit when you get dressed and keep your knees together when getting in and out of the car. Avoid stairs, going up them slowly sideways if you must. Don't do any squatting or yoga positions that involve separating or spreading the legs. You can substitute either of the positions below and still do the movements recommended for the upper body. When kneeling, use the position shown below instead of kneeling with your knees apart.

Plenty of warm baths and gentle swimming can be a relief, but avoid breaststroke which may strain the symphysis pubis, and take care getting in and out of the bath or pool. Wear well cushioned flat shoes. Be creative when you dress, tying a long scarf around your hips for support. For comfort, put a baby sheepskin under your hips or an "egg box" foam underlay under your bed sheet, and use a soft pillow to support your top leg when lying on your side. Contact a local SPD network (see p. 93) for advice.

Discuss your care in labour with your birth attendants to avoid greater separation of the legs than you can manage comfortably, and consider possible labour and birth positions such as lying on your side, kneeling on all fours, or immersion in warm water. Be especially careful of spreading the legs too wide if you have an epidural which may mask the pain. After birth, the first two weeks are crucial to a good recovery, so be careful to avoid strain at this time.

Place a pile of three or more cushions between your calves and under your pelvis so that you feel completely comfortable. Keep your knees together and your feet turned in toward the cushions. Use a scarf to tie the thighs together for support. Let your weight drop through your hips.

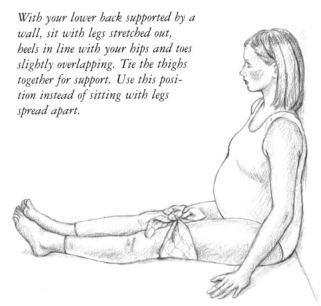

With your lower back supported by a wall, sit with legs stretched out, heels in line with your hips and toes slightly overlapping. Tie the thighs together for support. Use this position instead of sitting with legs spread apart.

Cramp

Muscle cramps are common in pregnancy and often occur as sudden spasms in the calves. Individual spasms only last a few minutes and may result from the weight you are carrying. They may also be caused by circulation changes or calcium deficiency.

Prevention Exercise regularly (see pp. 30-41) and make sure your diet contains sufficient calcium (see p. 25), or take a calcium and magnesium supplement. Do the exercise below regularly.

Professional treatment *Acupuncture* and *Osteopathy* Both these treatments can be effective in relieving cramp.

Self-help suggestions Immediately the cramp begins, massage and stretch the muscle by extending your heel and bringing your toes toward you. The exercise illustrated below may bring relief if done during a spasm; it may also help to prevent cramp. *Homeopathy* Dissolve four tablets of the tissue salt Magnesia phosphorica 6X in a small glass of warm water and sip when cramp occurs. *Herbalism* A decoction of cramp bark may be helpful. Simmer 28g (1oz) of the dried roots in 840ml (1½ pt) water for 20 minutes. Leave to cool, strain, and drink three glasses daily. *Shiatsu* Apply pressure to the point illustrated below to bring relief.

Exercise
Stand 30cm (12in) away from the wall. Bend your front knee and lean forward, with your arms on the wall. Keeping your back knee straight, move the foot as far back as you can without lifting the heel. Hold for a few seconds, dropping your weight into your back heel. Change legs. Repeat several times.

Shiatsu
Flex your right foot. Locate the point Liver 4 (LIV4) in the depression between the tendon and the inside ankle bone. Press for 5-7 seconds. Repeat 3 times.

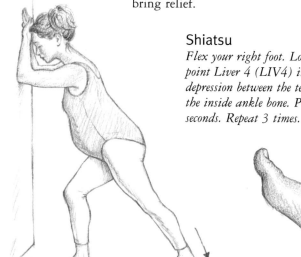

Nausea

Nausea, also known as "morning sickness", and mild vomiting are common symptoms in early pregnancy. You may experience feelings of nausea accompanied by tiredness and lethargy at different times of the day, but usually the symptoms will clear up by the end of the first three months. Occasionally, symptoms can continue throughout pregnancy, and may be more likely to do so if you are expecting twins. Severe vomiting that does not stop requires urgent medical attention.

Although the causes of nausea in pregnancy are not yet known, the following have been suggested as contributory factors: low blood sugar, low blood pressure, hormonal changes, emotional ambivalence about the pregnancy, food deficiency (in particular of vitamin B6 and iron), an excess of refined, spicy, or greasy foods, and pressure on the stomach from the growing uterus in the last few weeks of pregnancy.

Professional treatment *Homeopathy* There are several remedies which can be effective, so consultation with a homeopath is recommended. *Acupuncture, Psychotherapy*, and *Cranial osteopathy* These therapies may all be effective in relieving nausea. *Herbalism* Consultation with a herbalist is recommended since there is such a wide range of herbs that may be useful. Chamomile and wild yam root, for example, aid digestion and have a sedative effect, while balm and meadowsweet are soothing.

Self-help suggestions Listed below are some useful tips and natural remedies that may be helpful for nausea. If one remedy doesn't work, experiment with another.

Practise deep breathing, meditation, and yoga (see pp. 18-21 and 30-43) and try to take an hour's walk in the fresh air every day. Consider possible emotional causes and seek professional help if need be, or discuss your feelings with someone understanding.

A protein-rich snack eaten half an hour before you go to bed in the evening will help to ensure that your blood sugar level doesn't fall too low during the night. Try to remember to get up slowly out of bed and take your time in the morning. You may find a teaspoon of cider vinegar in a cup of warm water helpful first thing. An infusion of grated ginger root may bring relief if drunk while you are feeling nauseous. Increase the iron-rich foods in your diet (see p. 25) and, if you have no appetite, take 10 to 20g of vitamin B6 as a daily supplement.

Homeopathy For severe nausea, try Nux vomica 30C, Sepia 30C, or Ipecacuana 30C three times daily for five days, stopping earlier if symptoms start to improve. If there is no improvement, consult a homeopath. *Herbalism* Slippery elm tablets will soothe the digestive tract – take two with each meal or add the powder to your food. *Shiatsu* Applying pressure to the stomach meridian (see *Heartburn*, p. 88) or to the point PC6 (see *Anxiety*, p. 69) may alleviate symptoms. *Aromatherapy* Use essential oils of lavender, chamomile, and rose, either singly or combined, as a massage oil. You can also put a drop or two of one of these on a tissue and carry it with you.

Breakfast for morning sickness

Stay in bed for half an hour after waking and sip a herbal tea (see p. 63 for a list of herbal teas that aid digestion) with a few dry crackers or a glass of mineral water. Rise slowly, take some fresh fruit or fruit juice and breathe deeply in the open air. Half an hour later have a slice of wholegrain toast with yeast extract and a second cup of herbal tea.

Constipation

Constipation can become a problem during pregnancy since hormonal changes cause food to move more slowly through your digestive system. A poor diet lacking in fibre may be the cause, but stress, tension, and occasionally food allergy may also be contributory factors. Synthetic iron supplements, commonly prescribed in pregnancy, can also cause constipation (see *Anaemia*, p. 77 for alternatives).

Prevention Regular exercise (see pp. 30-43) and a diet which includes plenty of fresh vegetables, fruit, and whole, rather than refined, foods (see pp. 22-29), will help to ensure movement of food through your digestive system. Try to avoid eating too much red meat and make sure you are drinking enough fluids including herbal teas, fruit and vegetable juices, spring water, soups, and milkshakes in your diet. Drinking a cup of hot water or herbal tea when you first wake up may be helpful but, above all, try not to rush first thing in the morning – give yourself time to relax. When you feel the urge to defecate, try to respond immediately. Remember to breathe deeply and to relax and avoid straining when emptying your bowels. Adopting a squatting position before defecating will help to relax your bowel.

Professional treatment *Acupuncture* or *Shiatsu* Both these therapies will help to release blocked energy. *Homeopathy* Constitutional treatment (see p. 65) can be helpful. *Aromatherapy* Massage with essential oils may help chronic constipation.

Self-help suggestions Avoid the use of laxatives and increase your intake of fibre-rich foods, especially raw or lightly steamed green vegetables and fresh fruit. Reduce the amount of dairy products in your diet (see p. 27 for alternatives). The gluten in bread can clog up the intestines so try eating rice cakes or gluten-free bread instead. It's a good idea to add organic oat bran to your diet, but remember to drink plenty of fluids as well. For breakfast, try dried prunes or figs soaked in water overnight or drink ready-prepared prune juice.

Exercise regularly (see pp. 30-43) and take care to practise squatting daily. Massage your belly regularly (see p. 46), working in a clockwise direction and following the path of the large intestine. *Homeopathy* Take Nux Vomica 6X three times daily for up to a week. Stop if there is an improvement and repeat when needed; if symptoms fail to improve, consult a professional homeopath.

Heartburn

The hormones released during pregnancy soften the valve between the oesophagus and stomach. As a result, foods and gastric acids may back up, irritating the lining of the oesophagus and causing a feeling of pain and an acute burning sensation in the chest. Pressure on the stomach from the growing uterus may make the symptoms worse, especially during the later months. Heartburn usually occurs after meals, often as a result of combining the wrong foods or eating too quickly, but it can happen at any time and may follow an emotional upset.

Prevention Eat small meals at frequent intervals and aim to finish your evening meal at least two hours before going to bed. Take time over your meals, chewing your food well, and avoid lying down when relaxing after eating. Cut out spicy, greasy, sugary, acidic, or other foods that disagree with you and try not to drink with your meals as this dilutes the digestive juices. Sipping a herbal infusion of fennel after meals will aid digestion, but it is best to avoid stimulants such as tea and coffee.

Self-help suggestions Try alkaline foods such as yoghurt or milk to ease the burning. If these do not work, try mildly acidic foods such as orange, pineapple, or tomato juice. Papaya contains digestive enzymes and may be eaten fresh or in tablet form. Dried, salted umeboshi plums from Japan, available from health-food stores, are a great aid to digestion. A tea made from one cup of boiled water and one umeboshi plum can be flavoured with tamari and drunk hot or cold. An infusion of meadowsweet has a digestive, soothing effect. In cases of severe heartburn, eating proteins and carbohydrates separately at different times during the day may help to improve digestion. Vegetables may be combined with either proteins or carbohydrates, but fruit is best eaten at the beginning rather than at the end of a meal.

Practising the shoulder stretch and inner thigh stretch exercises on pages 39 and 41 may help to bring relief. *Herbalism* One teaspoon of slippery elm powder mixed with water or milk will neutralise the stomach. *Homeopathy* Take either Aresenicum 6C or Natrum phosphoricum 6C three times daily, stopping when symptoms start to improve. If there is no improvement, consult a homeopath. *Shiatsu* Apply pressure to the point PC6 (see *Anxiety*, p. 69) and ask your partner to shiatsu the stomach meridian as illustrated below.

Shiatsu

Helper: with your partner sitting on the floor with her back supported, place one hand on her upper thigh. Using the thumb of your other hand, shiatsu along the stomach meridian (shown). Concentrate on pressing the point Stomach 36 (ST36), located four fingers' width below the kneecap in the indentation on the outside of the shin bone.

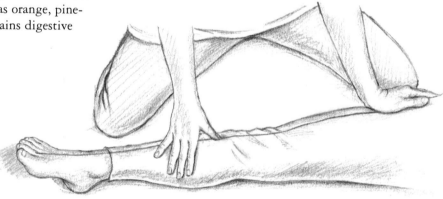

Diarrhoea

If you suffer an attack of diarrhoea, your stools will become loose and watery and you may experience abdominal pains and flatulence. Sudden attacks are usually short lived and are, more often than not, the body's means of ridding itself of an unwanted or infective substance. They may be brought on by gastric infection, food poisoning, pollutants, antibiotic treatment, an unbalanced diet, too much vitamin C or sugar, overeating, anxiety, or an emotional upset. In late pregnancy diarrhoea is common in the days approaching birth. Long-lasting attacks, however, can lead to nutritional deficiency and need to be taken seriously. They may be caused by an allergy, salmonella, aluminium cooking utensils, stress, or continual overeating.

Prevention Try to reduce the overall amount of sugar in your diet. When travelling, particularly in hot countries, drink bottled water and peel all fruit and vegetables; avoid canned, preserved, processed, or other foods that may be contaminated or contain pollutants or toxic substances.

Professional treatment *Homeopathy* A wide range of remedies is effective in treating diarrhoea, therefore it is advisable to consult a homeopath. *Acupuncture* This therapy may help to balance the energies in cases of chronic diarrhoea.

Self-help suggestions To prevent dehydration, drink plenty of fluids, including water and herbal teas. Miss a meal and then eat gentle foods, such as brown rice, lightly steamed vegetables, live yoghurt, or ripe bananas, for a day or two. *Herbalism* Make an infusion of peppermint and chamomile (see *caution*, p. 63) or fennel, using one teaspoon of each herb to two cups of boiling water. Drink frequently during attacks. *First-aid homeopathy* If you suffer from acute food poisoning accompanied by diarrhoea and vomiting, take Arsenicum 30C immediately and repeat the dosage every two hours. If there is no improvement, consult a homeopath. Since some forms of food poisoning involving toxins may be dangerous for the unborn child, it is important to inform your doctor at the onset of symptoms.

Bladder and kidney problems

Your kidneys work harder during pregnancy due to the increased volume of fluid circulating in the body, and the additional stress can make your urinary system more vulnerable to infection. The infection of the bladder, known as cystitis, is not uncommon in pregnancy and is accompanied by burning sensations on urination, frequent urges to urinate which bring little relief, and, sometimes, mild aching or cramp in the abdomen. Pyelitis, an infection of the kidneys, is more serious than cystitis and is indicated by tenderness or pain in the lower back, fever, lethargy, and headaches. If the symptoms of pyelitis are accompanied by blood in the urine, you may have haematuria. You should consult your doctor about any urinary infection and discuss alternative forms of treatment that you are considering.

You may also, while pregnant, experience temporary incontinence on laughing or sneezing. This occurs as a result of the relaxing effect of the hormones released at this time, and usually disappears after the birth.

Prevention Avoid junk foods, refined starches, sugar, coffee, tea, and also foods with a high acidic content; eat live natural yoghurt every day. Drink plenty of fluids: barley water and nettle tea are especially beneficial. To prevent irritation, wear cotton underwear, wash your genitals with water rather than soap. After intercourse, emptying your bladder, and washing with water only, may help to reduce the risk of infec-

tions. After going to the toilet, wipe from front to back and wash if possible. To avoid catching a chill on the bladder, wear warm clothes in cold weather.

Professional treatment For any infection of the urinary tract, you should either consult your doctor or an alternative therapist. Antibiotic treatment can be avoided provided obvious improvement follows alternative therapy. *Homeopathy* or *Acupuncture* Both are excellent therapies for acute and chronic problems of the urinary tract. *Herbalism* Herbs such as uva ursi and corn silk are potent diuretics with antibacterial properties that can be more effective than antibiotics. Consult a good herbalist since these powerful herbs need careful prescription. *Aromatherapy* This treatment can be effective in treating chronic cystitis.

Self-help suggestions Urinary infections can worsen rapidly so it is important to treat symptoms promptly. Avoid acid foods, including sugar, fruit, and fruit juice. Start by drinking a pint of spring water, taking some every half hour to flush out your system. Include cabbage, garlic, and leeks in your diet, and drink plenty of cranberry juice, which you can blend with a handful of fresh parsley. Barley water is good for urinary infections, and herb teas such as chamomile (see *caution,* p. 63), raspberry leaf in the last three months of pregnancy, and marshmallow may be helpful. You can also try taking 500g daily of vitamin C until symptoms improve.

Breech baby

When a baby is in the breech position, the head lies beneath the mother's ribs and the buttocks are positioned above the pelvis. Many babies are breech during pregnancy. The majority turn head down in the last few weeks, but some do so just before the birth. A number of babies remain in the breech position and can often be born vaginally without complications. However, routine intervention is usually recommended and if your baby is still in the breech position at 34 weeks, it is worth encouraging a turn by following the guidelines given below.

Prevention Walking for at least an hour a day may encourage your baby's head – the heaviest part of the body – to go down.

Professional treatment *Acupuncture* Consult an acupuncturist together with your partner so that you can learn how to do moxibustion treatment daily on the point on the little toe that connects with the uterus. This will help to stimulate the movement of the baby if done while you are in the position illus-

trated below. *Homeopathy* A single dose of Pulsatilla, in a high potency, may be effective but the dosage should be prescribed and the progress monitored by a homeopath as constitutional treatment (see p. 65) may be needed as well.

Self-help suggestions Massaging your belly in the position illustrated below may help your baby to turn. Alternatively, you can adopt the knee-chest position (see p. 40, pelvic floor exercise, position *b*). Before you start, find out from your midwife or obstetrician which way your baby is likely to turn so you can massage in the right direction. Use a massage oil and work with your hands intuitively. Results are not usually immediate but keep trying as your baby may turn at any time, even during labour. To prevent the breech engaging, avoid squatting.

If you suspect that your baby has turned, stop all treatments. Once the turn is confirmed, you can start squatting to encourage the head to engage.

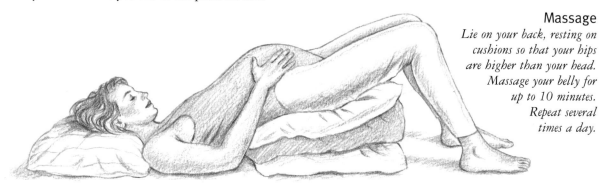

Massage
Lie on your back, resting on cushions so that your hips are higher than your head. Massage your belly for up to 10 minutes. Repeat several times a day.

Vaginal bleeding and miscarriage

Slight spotting is common in early pregnancy and may occur at times when your period would have been due, after making love, or as a result of a vaginal infection (see *Vaginal discharge*, p. 92) or cervical erosion. While it is unlikely to affect your baby or the pregnancy, it is wise to inform your doctor.

Heavier bleeding, especially if it is accompanied by pain or clots, needs immediate medical attention. Sometimes bleeding may stop after bedrest, with no harm to the foetus, and the pregnancy can continue;

in these instances, much can be done to strengthen the mother's potential to sustain the pregnancy. If bleeding escalates or is associated with cramps in the abdomen, a miscarriage generally follows. Up to 24 weeks may pass before the miscarriage actually takes place and while nothing will stop it if it is meant to happen, a lot can be done to prevent recurrence.

If miscarriage occurs in early pregnancy, it usually does so during the first ten to twelve weeks. An ultrasound scan may be used to confirm diagnosis.

A threatened miscarriage later on in pregnancy may result from a loose or "incompetent" cervix and can be prevented with a cervical stitch. Toward the end of pregnancy, blood-stained mucus may be a "show" and a sign that labour is imminent.

Preventing a threatened miscarriage Consult your doctor when bleeding occurs. Bedrest may be advised, and while there is no evidence that this prevents miscarriage, it is essential to take things easy. *Bach flower remedies* Rock Rose may be taken four times daily.

Preventing recurrent miscarriage Have a thorough gynaecological check-up to see if any obvious problems, such as an incompetent cervix, may have been the cause of your previous miscarriage. Spend the months before pregnancy improving your health generally, paying special attention to nutrition and exercise (see pp. 22-29 and 30-43). Avoid stimulants, alcohol, and cigarettes. *Herbalism* Black haw root bark, false unicorn root, or cramp bark may be taken to prevent miscarriage and help sustain the pregnancy, but they need to be prescribed by a herbalist. *Homeopathy* and *Acupuncture* These therapies may be used to correct imbalances prior to conception. *Counselling* If an emotional problem appears to be a contributory factor, arrange to see a therapist.

Treatment after miscarriage After miscarriage, a D & C (dilatation and curettage of the uterus) is usually recommended to remove any fragments from the uterus that might give rise to infection. This is done under anaesthetic in hospital. *Herbalism* A herbalist may prescribe herbs to clear the system and prevent infection after miscarriage. In some cases this treatment may be used as an alternative to D & C, but should only be taken in consultation with your doctor. *Acupuncture* This therapy can be used to help clear the uterus and aid its recover. *Counselling* Miscarriage can be a great shock and deeply upsetting. Give yourself time to mourn your loss before trying to conceive again. If problems persist, talking to a skilled counsellor may help.

Herpes

Recurring infections, sores, and blisters are characteristic symptoms of the herpes simplex virus, of which there are two types. If you are infected by type one, cold sores will appear on your lips or nostrils and will dry up, if left alone, in five to ten days. The sores are infectious and can be spread to the genitals by oral sex. The second type, known as genital herpes, is spread solely by sexual contact. The lesions, which appear on the vulva, in the vagina, or on the cervix, are painful to start with, later developing into blisters and finally infectious ulcers. While they will heal spontaneously, taking between 10 and 20 days to do so, the virus may remain dormant in the underlying nerves and, if reactivated, may cause another attack within weeks.

If the mother has open lesions at the time of birth, there is a risk that the baby may be infected while passing through the birth canal. A primary attack of herpes can cause serious damage to a newborn baby and, for this reason, birth by caesarean section is usually advised during a herpes outbreak. Risk to the baby diminishes in subsequent attacks since the mother develops antibodies to the virus. If the virus is present but dormant, vaginal birth can take place. After 36 weeks of pregnancy, tests by vaginal examination and viral culture are done weekly.

Professional treatment The drug Acyclovir is usually prescribed but, while it may speed up healing, it does not prevent recurrence. It may also be given to the baby after birth. *Herbalism* Herpes may be effectively treated with herbs but a skilled practitioner must be consulted. Wild oat, boxweed, burdock, garlic, and tincture of echinacae are known to be useful. *Homeopathy* Constitutional treatment (see p. 65) is recommended for helping to reduce the frequency and length of attacks. *Aromatherapy* Essential oils of lavender or tea tree can be helpful, but it is essential to consult a skilled aromatherapist. *Acupuncture* Regular acupuncture treatment will help to relieve stress and fatigue.

Self-help suggestions Try to avoid stressful situations and rest a good deal. Take a B complex vitamin supplement, and avoid tea, coffee, and sugar. *Herbalism* Ask a herbalist to make up a cream of dwarf nettle and calendula to relieve pain locally. Clean lesions in a sitting bath, made by adding a strong cup of chamomile tea to a bowl of warm water containing 10 drops of calendula tincture. *Homeopathy* Herpes type one can be treated with Natrum muriaticum 30C or Rhus toxicodendron 30C, taken three times daily for three days.

Thrush

Thrush is a common fungus, also known as yeast, monilla, or candida, that is normally present in the vagina. If the ecological balance of the vagina is disturbed, however, it can overgrow, causing redness, itching, and burning, and a flaky white, cheesy discharge. Outbreaks are common in pregnancy and, occasionally, become chronic. The baby may pick up the infection during birth, and while neo-natal thrush can be easily treated, it is preferable if the infection is cleared up before the birth.

Thrush may be caused by poor diet (particularly overconsumption of refined sugary foods), stress, anaemia, tiredness, use of antibiotics, or infection through sexual contact. A high blood sugar content, previous use of the pill, and the vaginal acidity that is commonly associated with pregnancy, may also be contributory factors.

Prevention Eat a wholesome, balanced diet (see pp. 22-29), eliminating acidic or sugary foods. Sleep and rest whenever you feel the need and try to reduce stress in your environment. Use homeopathic calendula soap rather than other types that may be too alkaline, and wash your genital area with your hand rather than a cloth. Always wipe from front to back. Avoid vaginal sprays and bubble baths. Tight trousers or nylon tights should not be worn since thrush will thrive in a warm, dark, airless environment. Either wear loose cotton underwear or none at all until the infection has cleared. Always wash and dry your swimsuit after use.

Professional treatment Your doctor may prescribe an anti-fungal pessary for you and a cream for your partner. To begin with this treatment may eradicate symptoms, but persistent use can lead to chronic thrush as the fungus becomes desensitized. *Homeopathy* This treatment can be very effective. *Acupuncture* This therapy may be used to strengthen the body's natural resistance to infection. *Herbalism* Consult a good herbalist about herbs that will combat infection. Infusions of herbs such as fennel, cornflower, or cleavers are helpful and may be prescribed.

Self-help suggestions Follow the preventive guidelines outlined above. Eat plenty of fresh garlic and live yoghurt, and add pure unrefined olive oil to your salads. Before going to sleep, insert a few teaspoons of live yoghurt into your vagina using your fingers, a teaspoon, a tampon, or a vaginal applicator. The live bacteria in the yoghurt will multiply and consume the thrush. Wash out your vagina in the bath the following morning, using your fingers, and repeat the treatment daily until symptoms improve. You can also try adding a few tablespoons of bicarbonate of soda to your bath water to reduce acidity. *Herbalism* To calm itching, apply a chamomile cream to the vulva several times a day or use a sitting bath of strong chamomile tea. Alternatively, wash the vulva with chamomile tea containing ten drops of calendula tincture. *Aromatherapy* The addition of ten drops of tea tree oil to your bath water is very helpful to ease symptoms and reduce thrush. *Homeopathy* Alternate Borax 30C and Candida 30C every three hours for three days.
Caution: do not use vaginal douches during pregnancy; sitting baths make a good alternative. Avoid sexual penetration during treatment for thrush.

Vaginal discharge

Vaginal secretions increase during pregnancy and may have a different smell and taste. If a discharge is white, yellow, or greenish in colour, or if there is an unpleasant odour or irritation, you should consult your doctor and obtain an accurate diagnosis of the cause of the disorder.

Professional treatment *Homeopathy, Herbalism,* or *Acupuncture* These therapies are used successfully to treat a variety of vaginal infections. It is advisable to go to your doctor for further tests a few weeks after the end of treatment to ensure that the infection has cleared up completely.

Self-help suggestions Pay attention to diet (see pp. 22-29), avoiding sugary and acidic foods, and get plenty of rest. *Homeopathy* The tissue salt Natrum phosphoricum 6X taken three times daily for a week will help to stabilize the acid/alkaline balance in your body and clear any discharge.

Author's acknowledgements (first edition)
My gratitude to the following practitioners for their help and advice; Miranda Castro, Judith Fogler (osteopathy), Elise Johnson (shiatsu), Beatrice Linhares (herbalism), Jan Resnick (acupuncture). My thanks also to Carole Eliott, Judith Fogler, Caroline Guy, Haya Oakley, Mina Semyon, Norman Stannard, Lolly Stirk, Mary Stewart, and Peter Walker, and to the mothers who modelled for artwork and photographs: Sharon Bannister, Silvana Calzavara, Susan Duffy, Sylvia Robinson, and Vicky de Wolfe. Finally I would like to thank Dr Yehudi Gordon for checking the manuscript, and the team at Gaia Books for their help.

Publisher's acknowledgements (first edition)
Gaia would like to thank the following: Lucy Su for her gentle and sensitive illustrations, Fausto Dorelli for his striking photography, Joss Pearson for advice and support, Lucy Lidell for initial work on the project, Dr Yehudi Gordon and Dr Richard Donze for checking the manuscript, Patrick Nugent for art direction, Sara Matthews for her sound design judgement, Rosanne Hooper and Jonathan Hilton for their invaluable editorial guidance, Susan Walby for her production expertise, Leslie Gilbert for her meticulous coding, Robin Hayward for professional advice, Lynette Beckford, Penny Cowdry, and all the expectant mothers and toddlers who posed as photographic models.